D1509095

Implications of Disaster Preparedness for Nursing

Editor

DEBORAH J. PERSELL

NURSING CLINICS
OF NORTH AMERICA

www.nursing.theclinics.com

Consulting Editor
STEPHEN D. KRAU

December 2016 • Volume 51 • Number 4

ELSEVIER

1600 John F. Kennedy Boulevard • Suite 1800 • Philadelphia, Pennsylvania, 19103-2899

http://www.theclinics.com

NURSING CLINICS OF NORTH AMERICA Volume 51, Number 4
December 2016 ISSN 0029-6465, ISBN-13: 978-0-323-47744-4

Editor: Kerry Holland
Developmental Editor: Casey Jackson

Nursing Clinics of North America (ISSN 0029-6465) is published quarterly by Elsevier Inc., 360 Park Avenue South, New York, NY 10010-1710. Months of issue are March, June, September, and December. Periodicals postage paid at New York, NY and additional mailing offices. Subscription price per year is, $155.00 (US individuals), $447.00 (US institutions), $275.00 (international individuals), $545.00 (international institutions), $220.00 (Canadian individuals), $545.00 (Canadian institutions), $100.00 (US students), and $135.00 (international students). To receive student/resident rate, orders must be accompanied by name of affiliated institution, date of term, and the signature of program/residency coordinator on institution letterhead. Orders will be billed at individual rate until proof of status is received. Foreign air speed delivery is included in all *Clinics* subscription prices. All prices are subject to change without notice. **POSTMASTER:** Send address changes to *Nursing Clinics*, Elsevier Health Sciences Division, Subscription Customer Service, 3251 Riverport Lane, Maryland Heights, MO 63043. **Customer Service: Telephone: 1-800-654-2452** (U.S. and Canada); **1-314-447-8871 (outside U.S. and Canada). Fax: 1-314-447-8029. E-mail: journalscustomerservice-usa@elsevier.com** (for print support) and **journalsonlinesupport-usa@elsevier.com** (for online support).

Nursing Clinics of North America is covered in EMBASE/Excerpta Medica, MEDLINE/PubMed (Index Medicus), Social Sciences Citation Index, Current Contents, ASCA, Cumulative Index to Nursing, RNdex Top 100, and Allied Health Literature and International Nursing Index (INI).

Printed in the United States of America.

Contributors

CONSULTING EDITOR

STEPHEN D. KRAU, PhD, RN, CNE
Associate Professor, Vanderbilt University School of Nursing, Nashville, Tennessee

EDITOR

DEBORAH J. PERSELL, PhD, RN, APN
Professor; Program Director, Regional Center for Disaster Preparedness Education, College of Nursing and Health Professions, Arkansas State University, Jonesboro, Arkansas

AUTHORS

ROBERT C. BEAUCHAMP, BSN, RN, CEN, EMT-P
Radiation Emergency Assistance Center/Training Site (REAC/TS), Oak Ridge Associated Universities, Oak Ridge, Tennessee

SUZANNE M. BOSWELL, PhD, MSN, RN, CCRA
Graduate, University of Tennessee, Knoxville, Tennessee

MARY CASEY-LOCKYER, RN, MHS, CCRN
American Red Cross, Washington, DC

BRENT COX, DM, CHEP
Assistant Professor, Regional Center for Disaster Preparedness Education, College of Nursing and Health Professions, Arkansas State University, Jonesboro, Arkansas

SHARON L. FARRA, RN, PhD, CNE
Assistant Professor, College of Nursing and Health, Wright State University, Dayton, Ohio

PATRICIA FROHOCK HANES, PhD, MSN, MAEd, MS-DPEM, RN, CNE
Professor, Azusa Pacific University School of Nursing, Azusa, California

DEBORAH H. KIM, APRN, MSN, CHEP
Senior Research Scientist, Division of Health and Consumer Solutions/Medical Readiness and Response, Battelle Memorial Institute, New York, New York

LAUREN M. OPPIZZI, MSN, RN
University of Tennessee College of Nursing, Knoxville, Knoxville, Tennessee

DEBORAH J. PERSELL, PhD, RN, APN
Professor; Program Director, Regional Center for Disaster Preparedness Education, College of Nursing and Health Professions, Arkansas State University, Jonesboro, Arkansas

FELECIA M. RIVERS, PhD, RN
Army Nurse Corps; Adjunct Assistant Professor, Arkansas State University, Jonesboro, Arkansas

STASIA E. RUSKIE, PhD, RN
Albuquerque, New Mexico

SHERRILL J. SMITH, RN, PhD, CNL, CNE
Associate Professor, Assistant Dean for Undergraduate Programs, College of Nursing and Health, Wright State University, Dayton, Ohio

SUSAN SPERAW, PhD, RN
Retired, University of Tennessee College of Nursing, Knoxville, Signal Mountain, Tennessee

JANICE SPRINGER, DNP, RN, PHN
Public Health Consultant; Division Disability Integration Advisor, Disaster Health Services, American Red Cross, Washington, DC

Contents

Health care emergency preparedness has undergone significant changes since the first widespread distribution of federal funds occurred in 2002. Prior to the development of the Health Resources and Service Administration Bioterrorism Preparedness grant, support to hospitals and public health was limited to smaller regional preparedness programs such as the Chemical Stockpile Emergency Preparedness Program. Measurable progress with both the hospital preparedness program and public health emergency preparedness requires development of partnerships, establishment of coalitions, development of measurable objectives, and a community willingness to work together to solve complex preparedness problems.

As the largest profession of health care providers, nurses are an integral component of disaster response. Having clearly delineated competencies and developing training to acquire those competencies are needed to ensure nurses are ready when disasters occur. This article provides a review of nursing and interprofessional disaster competencies and development of a new interprofessional disaster certification. An overview of a standardized disaster training program, the National Disaster Health Consortium, is provided as an exemplar of a competency-based interprofessional disaster education program.

US nurses are not prepared for the altered conditions of the disaster environment, nor has the context of providing disaster nursing care been a focus of disaster research. Using an existential phenomenologic approach, US nurses described the "not normal" conditions of the disaster environment they experienced as physically and emotionally challenging, because of the reduced infrastructural capabilities, unfamiliar patient

Major nursing organizations support disaster education for nurses. It is essential for nurses to recognize their roles in each phase of the disaster cycle: mitigation, preparedness, response, and recovery. Skills learned in the US federal all-hazards approach to disasters can then be adapted to more specific disasters, such as wildfires, and issues affecting health care. Nursing has an important role in each phase of the disaster cycle.

From the time of Clara Barton, Red Cross nursing has had a key role in the care and support of persons affected by disasters in the United States. Hurricane Katrina and other events brought to light the need for a shelter model that was inclusive of the whole community, including persons with disabilities, at-risk and vulnerable populations, and children. From an intake process to a nursing model for assessment, an evidence-guided process informed a systematic approach for a registered nurse–led model of care.

Incidents involving the release of hazardous materials challenge medical providers with safely, quickly, and correctly removing contaminants from the victim. While doing so, the safety of the first receiver, current patients, bystanders, as well as the victim all have to be considered. Key challenges with hospital decontamination include, but are not limited to, selection of team members, training protocols, employee turnover, and funding. Best practices, based on the available literature and evidence, include administration buy-in and support; strong policy and procedure documentation; equipment maintenance programs; and team member recruitment, retention, and education.

Lack of understanding about the basic nature of radiation exposure and contamination may lead to unreasonable fear in nursing staff. A brief review of a well-known case shows that in general, both the public and health care providers are radiophobic. Studies have shown that the level of fear correlates inversely with an understanding of radiation. This article explores underlying principles of ionizing radiation and their application in patient management. Reality based, scientifically accurate information along with practical suggestions can free health care providers from unreasonable fear of victims of a radiation accident.

In August 2005, the United States experienced one of the most catastrophic and costly disasters in its history: Hurricane Katrina. Faith-based

Organizations (FBOs) made a major contribution to the response and recovery efforts. Whereas the activities and skill sets of FBOs vary, their core missions are very similar: they want to provide hope. As a concept, hope has been purported to be essential for health and well-being, is viewed as multidimensional and a life force, as well as is highly individualized. This mixed methods study used interviews of the phenomenology tradition and the Herth Hope Index.

NURSING CLINICS OF NORTH AMERICA

FORTHCOMING ISSUES

March 2017
Advances in Oncology Nursing
Margaret Barton-Burke, *Editor*

June 2017
Fluids and Electrolytes
Joshua Squiers, *Editor*

September 2017
Geriatric Nursing
Sally Miller and Jennifer Kim, *Editors*

RECENT ISSUES

September 2016
Palliative Care
James C. Pace and Dorothy Wholihan, *Editors*

June 2016
Psychiatric Mental Health Nursing
Deborah Antai-Otong, *Editor*

March 2016
Pharmacology Updates
Jennifer Wilbeck, *Editor*

ISSUE OF RELATED INTEREST

Emergency Medicine Clinics of North America, February 2015 (Volume 33, Issue 1)
Management of Hazardous Material Emergencies
Stephen W. Borron and Ziad Kazzi, *Editors*

Foreword

Disaster Planning, Preparedness, Mitigation, Response, and Recovery: A Call for All Nurses to Action

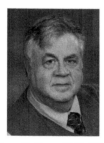

Stephen D. Krau, PhD, RN, CNE
Consulting Editor

One need only look at the Emergency Events Data Base created by the World Health Organization and the Belgian government to identify an alarming increase in natural disasters over the last decade. Natural disasters are those catastrophic events caused by forces of nature, which include a large variety of classifications. Predictions are these trends will increase globally as there are many practical and theoretical factors that continue to exacerbate these occurrences.

In addition to disasters that are created by nature are the disasters created by humans. Man-made disasters are those that are caused by human error or intent, or human negligence. These can include civil unrest and terrorism, fires, toxic emissions, chemical or biological warfare, and nuclear events. There remains some controversy over the impact of global warming on the occurrence of disasters. There is no question as to the increasing trends that can occur at any time and any place.

Historically, nurses have served as first responders to disasters even at the risk of personal sacrifice. Those nurses educated and trained in disaster care are postured to respond in effective and rehearsed manner. It is those nurses who are not in typical emergency roles that may be called upon to respond. This issue of *Nursing Clinics of North America* is a step in opening doors to discussions and exchange of ideas not only among nurses prepared for emergency disaster situations but also for those who are in other areas of nursing that might be called upon to respond. This issue provides thought-provoking information and a call to action as nurses consider all

Nurs Clin N Am 51 (2016) xi–xii
http://dx.doi.org/10.1016/j.cnur.2016.09.002
0029-6465/16/© 2016 Published by Elsevier Inc.

phases of the Disaster Cycle: Planning, Preparedness, Mitigation, Response, and Recovery.

Stephen D. Krau, PhD, RN, CNE
Vanderbilt University School of Nursing
461 21st Avenue South
Nashville, TN 37240, USA

E-mail address:
steve.krau@vanderbilt.edu

Preface

Implications of Disaster Preparedness for Nursing

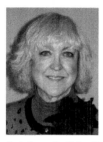

Deborah J. Persell, PhD, RN, APN
Editor

This issue of the *Nursing Clinics of North America* is devoted to disaster nursing. With ever-increasing frequency, nurses participate in all aspects of the disaster cycle (planning, preparedness, mitigation, response, and recovery). The articles contained in this issue reflect the broad scope of disaster nursing. Deborah Kim offers a historical overview and comprehensive study of statutory and regulatory processes that provide a foundation to understanding the response to disasters that impact nurses every day. Drs Farra and Smith build on this by framing the role and expectation of competencies in disaster nursing. They provide an excellent exemplar that may lead to a new certification in disaster nursing.

There is an emphasis on qualitative research in the issue. This is deliberate and intended to provide new understanding of the nurses' experiences in disaster. Their stories are powerful and challenge what we believe about nurses and the clients or patients served in times of disaster. Dr Ruskie begins by demonstrating the impact of the disaster environment on individual nurses. Dr Boswell examines the moral incongruence nurses experience as the circumstances of disaster nursing refuse to "fit" routine decision making. Then, Drs Oppizzi and Speraw present powerful evidence suggesting that not all help provided during disasters is understood, equitable, or helpful. The personal and professional impact of active duty military nurses being deployed to civilian disaster response is significant and demonstrated by Dr Rivers.

Wildfires present a unique threat to health and are frequently viewed as a firefighter and emergency management event, not a nursing one. Dr Hanes takes us inside the threat and demonstrates the vulnerabilities to communities, the impact on population and individual health as well as the implications for nurses providing care to victims of wildfires.

Almost all threats hold the potential for contamination. The nuances of medical decontamination are poorly understood and represent a challenge to the health care workforce. Dr Cox details the current state of medical decontamination, discusses

Nurs Clin N Am 51 (2016) xiii–xiv
http://dx.doi.org/10.1016/j.cnur.2016.09.001
0029-6465/16/© 2016 Published by Elsevier Inc.

the challenges of being a first receiver of a contaminated patient, and offers evidence-based processes for medical decontamination for chemicals. This is followed by an even more misunderstood and feared radiation decontamination event. Rob Beauchamp skillfully guides us through principles of radiation, contamination, and decontamination of this unique threat.

It is common for disasters to result in the need for shelters to be established. The Red Cross has much experience in setting up shelters and requires nursing presence in each shelter. Dr Springer and Mary Lockyer share a protocol to quickly identify health issues in shelters.

Finally, the concept of hope is well represented in nursing literature. The significance of hope in the context of disaster is demonstrated by the mixed methods research of Dr Persell. In the midst of devastating disaster conditions, hope can be a life-sustaining force for the nurse and those for whom the nurse cares.

Deborah J. Persell, PhD, RN, APN
Regional Center for Disaster Preparedness Education
College of Nursing and Health Professions
Arkansas State University
105 North Caraway
PO Box 910
State University (Jonesboro), AR 72467, USA

E-mail address:
dpersell@astate.edu

Emergency Preparedness and the Development of Health Care Coalitions
A Dynamic Process

Deborah H. Kim, APRN, MSN, CHEP

KEYWORDS

- Health care coalition • Patient surge • Resilience • Emergency preparedness

KEY POINTS

- Federally funded Hospital Preparedness Program and the Public Health Emergency Preparedness Programs have become aligned.
- Preparing for medical surge in the hospital and community is difficult.
- Health care coalitions can enhance health system resilience.
- Hospital evacuation is difficult to plan for and to carry out.
- Emergency preparedness requirements have changed and have additional requirements as defined by the Centers for Medicaid and Medicare Services (CMS).

INTRODUCTION

Health care emergency preparedness and the importance of a well-rehearsed, coordinated response have never been more important to the health security of a community or to the nation. Whether it is the threat of terrorism, climate change resulting in flooding, or a new virus for which there is no cure, the health care system will be on the forefront of response. The ability of hospitals, health care systems and the emergency medical system (EMS) to quickly transfer patients, be ready for critically injured people, provide medical counter measures (MCMs), or to initiate just-in-time training to staff to keep people safe is always uppermost for any first responder or hospital first receiver.[1] The role of the nurse in emergency preparedness may not always be visible. Historically, the nurse has not only been the bedside caregiver but a leader in seeing the larger picture when it applies to the hospital or health care community. Nursing process involves collaboration, which is the foundation for effective emergency preparedness and the process of emergency management.[2]

Division of Health and Consumer Solutions/Medical Readiness and Response, Battelle Memorial Institute, New York, NY, USA
E-mail address: deborahhkim3@gmail.com

Nurs Clin N Am 51 (2016) 545–554
http://dx.doi.org/10.1016/j.cnur.2016.07.013
0029-6465/16/© 2016 Elsevier Inc. All rights reserved.

nursing.theclinics.com

HOSPITAL EMERGENCY PREPAREDNESS: HISTORY

Hospital emergency preparedness is not a new idea. Hospitals as part of cities and towns in the 1930s were involved with civil defense programs after learning of the pre-war activities in Europe. World War II civil defense efforts and later on in the 1950s continued as communities prepared for potential nuclear attacks, and hospitals prepared for mass casualties. One the earliest hospital evacuation exercises took place in Portland, Oregon, in 1955 as part of Operation Green Light, a civil defense exercise.[3]

Historically, hospitals crafted a disaster plan with a trauma or mass casualty focus. The disaster plan began in the emergency department (ED) and ended when the patient was admitted to the hospital, died, or was discharged. Leadership for the hospital disaster plan was often carried out by nurses and other hospital leaders including: the nurse manager in the ED, trauma nurse coordinator, ED medical director, trauma medical director, hospital safety officer, or the hospital facility manager. Hospital EDs maintained a supply of medical surgical supplies, triage tags, and premade patient charts. The hospital engineering staff checked the emergency generator as part of the requirements for facility management, and load bank tests were carried out. Training on the hospital disaster plan usually occurred once a year and included a review of specific processes through table-top exercises. The greatest effort for training usually occurred in the ED. It is important to note that things have now changed.

Hospitals have coordinated as needed with local and state health departments, particularly in the development of large systems such as Emergency Medical Services for Children (EMSC), developing resources for large-scale mass emergency pediatric critical care,[4] emergency medical systems (EMS), and state trauma systems. Public health departments have historically taken the lead with viral or bacterial diseases that have had the potential to impact large numbers of the population such as norovirus, polio, varicella, rubella, meningitis, foodborne illness, and influenza. Highly virulent public health threats including Ebola virus disease (EVD), pandemic influenza, severe acute respiratory syndrome (SARS), and Zika virus disease require close coordination of both hospitals and public health officials to ensure accurate case counts, worker protection, protocols for testing, processing of laboratory samples, and early identification of those with the disease.

The National Defense Authorization Act for FY 1997 saw the allocation of funds aimed at enhancing domestic preparedness capabilities to respond to a weapons of mass destruction (WMD) incident. This act provided training to first responders (police and fire department) and to assist with the formation of metropolitan medical strike teams (MMSTs). WMD incidents are defined as terrorist-driven biological, chemical, radiological, and nuclear terrorism events. Training was provided to the 120 largest cities in the United States (by 1990 census data). The training, funded by the US Department of Defense (DoD), leveraged interagency coordination between US Federal Emergency Management Agency (FEMA), the US Department of Justice, and the DoD. Hospitals or the personnel responsible for emergency preparedness were not specifically included for training.[5] High-profile events such as the Atlanta Summer Olympics (1996) and the Salt Lake City Winter Olympics (2002) provided additional federal funds for first responders, public safety, and the development of patient care protocols. Hospitals may also choose to part of the National Medical Disaster System (NDMS). NDMS is a federal program comprised of partnerships between the Department of Health and Human Services (DHHS), the Department of Homeland Security (DHS) and the Department of Veteran's Affairs (VA). NDMS hospitals provide internal surge capability for disasters occurring in the United States, and also provide support to the military and VA hospital systems in providing casualty care for injured personnel from overseas conflicts.

EARLY FEDERAL SUPPORT FOR HOSPITAL PREPAREDNESS: THE CHEMICAL STOCKPILE EMERGENCY PREPAREDNESS PROGRAM

Training with other competing health care organizations to enhance hospital emergency preparedness has only recently come to light as an important cornerstone to US health care system resiliency. Although difficult to believe, the same foundations have existed within the Chemical Stockpile Emergency Preparedness Program (CSEPP) for over 20 years. Prior to development of CSEPP in 1985, there was little if any financial support for hospitals to develop/test disaster plans, purchase personal protective/decontamination, or drill with community partners.

CSEPP is a regional/state-based program that provided funding to hospitals and communities whose nearby neighbor includes a US Army military base that stored chemical weapons. Congress passed legislation in 1983 that required the US chemical weapons stockpile to be destroyed, and that maximum assistance was to be provided to the communities who were adjacent to the storage depots. Chemical weapon storage areas, also referred to as storage depots, were originally placed during the 1940s in remote areas, away from population centers. The chemical stockpiles contained munitions of either blister or nerve agents. They were located in Alabama, Arkansas, Indiana, Illinois, Maryland, Oregon, Washington, and Utah. Of the original 10 sites, 2 sites remain active, Pueblo, Colorado, and Lexington, Kentucky, and anticipate agent destruction beginning in 2016. Funding for the CSEPP is a cooperative grant process, funded through DoD (US Army) with support from FEMA. Assistance is provided during the time that stockpile destruction facilities are constructed and through the end of chemical agent destruction.[6]

Each community (including hospitals) developed plans and capabilities several areas, called "Benchmarks":

- Alert and notification include the various public communication devices that notify both military or the community of the release of a chemical agent. Notification devices include sirens, tone alert radios, and highway reader boards (electronic signs).
- Automated data processing means the ability of critical monitoring systems for an unintended chemical agent release to be seen by military base leaders, public information officers, and community leaders.
- Communications are comprised of interoperative, functional information-sharing systems that link the military on post leaders (base commander and support staff) with state leaders, local community leaders, response agencies (police, fire, and EMS), and citizens. Communication systems include video teleconferencing, portable radios, fax machines, cell phones, radio/television studios or broadcast, and telephones.
- Coordinated plans include emergency preparedness plans that are specific for each state, military installation, and for communities closest to the storage depot/chemical weapons destruction facility. These locations are at greatest risk should an off post release of chemical agent occur though a spill or airborne means. Coordinated plans involve identification of specific geographic zones. These locations are either the closest to the military base (therefore at greatest risk) or are further away (lower risk). These locations are referred to as the immediate response zones (IRZ) and the protective action zones (PAZ).
- Decontamination is the process of removing a chemical agent (nerve agent or blister agent) from clothing, skin or hard surface, or through washing with soap and water. The use of bottled bleach or a bleach solution is not recommended for skin, hair, or body surface decontamination.

- The emergency operations center (EOC) is a physical location that contains electronic communication devices such as radios, computer support, and telephones that coordinates a response to a disaster event. CSEPP-supported EOCs also contain computer systems that monitor the accidental release of a chemical agent off the military base (note—a release of chemical agent off post into the community has not occurred during the agent destruction or storage process).
- The term exercises refers to a program of testing and evaluation of the community (state and local governments, first responders, hospital personnel) to respond to an off post release of chemical agent. This includes coordination of messages (alert and notification), evacuation to a different location, setting up decontamination areas, decontamination of potential agent exposure, medical care, and other tasks.
- Personnel include various supportive roles for the program including program coordinators, planners, and public affairs/public information officers.
- The CSEPP program provides funding for the purchase of personal protective equipment (PPE) that is intended to protect workers from exposure to military chemical agent during the process of decontamination (removal of agent from the skin, clothing, or hair). Chemically resistant suits, gloves, boots, and powered air purifying respirators (PAPRS) are provided. The level of protection in the community is at US Occupational Safety and Health Agency (OSHA) level C. Higher levels of worker protection/PPE are in place on the military installation, and at the first responder level (fire department). As required by both US Army and OSHA regulations, extensive training is required before personnel can put on PPE and use the equipment either in a simulated or real-world situation.
- Education and training programs should be consistent with FEMA, state, and local areas. A training plan (for off post jurisdictions) and US Army certification requirements (for on post installations) is developed, and maintained proficiency of emergency services providers/responders, and CSEPP staff (as defined and measured by CSEPP guidance) is developed and presented on a scheduled basis.
- Medical support is comprised of a medical program for off post medical preparation and response to a CSEPP incident/accident. The medical support program includes several elements:
  - Medical guidance that addresses the relevant aspects of worker protection and patient care for individuals potentially exposed to a chemical agent release
  - Medical training for personnel to perform specified patient care activities, such as screening, triage, treatment, decontamination, transport, disposition, and patient tracking
  - Medical emergency operations that are in accordance with CSEPP guidance and federal, state, local, and generally accepted standards for patient care and worker protection
  - Coordinated medical plans and procedures, as appropriate, with the CSEPP alert and notification system, the Joint Information Center (JIC), and the Joint Information System (JIS)
  - Ensure that medical personnel participate in community response and recovery planning and community-based exercise and evaluation programs
  - Public awareness—multi-media information that is provided to the general public related to what chemical agents are stored on the military base, the processes of agent destruction, and information related to planning for family/individual shelter in place or evacuation, should it become necessary.

Participation in the CSEPP program is a commitment from both public health partners (local and state) and hospitals[7] in the state where the stockpile is located. A memorandum of understanding (MOU) is executed, which details the responsibilities of both the hospital as well as government partners. MOU hospitals receive supplies of medical countermeasures (autoinjectors of atropine and pralidoxime) if the stockpile site contains nerve agent. Decontamination supplies and PPE purchases are also funded. A comprehensive medical management course is offered to all CSEPP health care partners (hospital and prehospital). The all hazards course contains additional information on agent identification, decontamination, personal protective equipment use, medical countermeasure administration, incident command structure, alert/notification strategies, chemical casualty patient surge, and patient casualty medical management.

Prior to the development of the role of hospital emergency manager, nurses who were leaders in MOU hospital EDs or the hospital safety officers were often responsible for developing specific hospital plans as part of their participation in CSEPP. They formed collaborative relationships with other hospitals in order to learn from each other and plan for potential chemical casualties. These early collaborations/ coalitions were called integrated process teams (IPTs). The medical IPT included prehospital providers, specifically fire department hazardous materials teams (HAZ-MATs), physicians, and nurses. HAZMAT teams assisted in development of the requirements that would be needed for receiving potentially contaminated patients. Public health program managers served as liaisons between state emergency management, FEMA and US Army points of contact. IPTs established performance measures used not only for exercise evaluation, but also for planning guidance.

An evaluation of each CSEPP community's level of readiness occurs each year. Each CSEPP MOU hospital and its community partners participate in a full-scale annual exercise. Evaluators external to the community evaluate the ability of the community to respond to a chemical agent event both at on post (US Army storage location) and off post (community) locations. Hospital triage, decontamination, incident command system (ICS), implementation, and patient management are evaluated. Prehospital care and participation of first responders are also evaluated as part of the continuum of victim care. Exercise response outcomes (EROs) are used to measure progress in meeting specific objectives, and can be followed over the length of time that the program is in place for each community. Annual exercises reveal strengths and weakness. For example, new staff at a hospital may be unfamiliar with how to put on PPE, set up decontamination sites, or communicate with state and local leaders. Exercises teach and test. Within the medical environment, following requirements for dealing with hazardous materials is particularly important, and something that is closely evaluated each year. As with any disaster exercise or event, a prior understanding of the emergency operations plan, special procedures, or the use of equipment not used on a daily basis is vital. Safety issues, whether for simulated victims or people performing decontamination, are closely scrutinized. For example, stores of medical countermeasures (nerve agent antidote kits) are counted annually as well as medication expiration dates. One of the greatest challenges in the CSEPP program is personnel turnover, and loss of institutional memory, meaning a key person leaves an organization who knew where everything was located and how the procedure was to be carried out. The evaluation process at a hospital site identifies actions or plans that go well or need correction. This establishes a continuous quality improvement cycle whose elements can be measured over time.

Exercise Response Outcomes

Identification of areas in need of improvement or recognizing a process that reflects best process is inherent in the CSEPP program's exercise and evaluation process.

The metrics for evaluating exercise performance (EROs) have been developed for several areas:

ERO 1 prevention and preparedness—does the community/state/hospital have an emergency operations plan and process? How often is the plan updated? Is the update documented? Is the plan followed?

ERO 2 emergency assessment—has there been a release of agent? Where is it located? What has been released? Who is in danger?

ERO 3 emergency management—organization and response of state and local officials who plan for disasters

ERO 4 chemical agent identification (CAI)/hazard mitigation—do personnel know how to operate chemical agent detection equipment and interpret the results?

ERO 5 protection—are communities at the greatest risk notified in a timely manner? Are people/animals evacuated or sheltered in place?

ERO 6 victim care[a]—this is where public health, EMS, and hospital performance is measured (see descriptions listed previously under the benchmark section for medical support). Victim care has also been extended to include pets and livestock considerations.

ERO 7 emergency public information—how quickly does emergency information get shared with the community regarding a potential release of chemical agent?

ERO 8 remediation/recovery—what processes are followed to determine it is safe for people to return to their home or community? What additional steps need to be taken?

Hospital requirements such as those described in the US Joint Commission (JC) Emergency Preparedness standards are used as benchmarks when evaluating hospital performance. Each CSEPP exercise includes the required elements from the US

The US National Disaster Medical System (NDMS) is a federally coordinated system designed to supplement the integrated national medical response to a disaster in the form of personnel, teams, supplies, and equipment. NDMS is also involved with patient movement from a disaster site to unaffected areas of the United States, and provision of medical care at participating hospitals in unaffected areas. There are several things to note concerning NDMS:

- Part of the US Department of Health and Human Services (DHHS)—Office of Preparedness and Response

- Part of Emergency Support Function #8 (ESF8)

- Assists with provision of medical care at times of disaster

- Supports the US Department of Veteran Affairs in caring for casualties from war after they are transported back to the United States

Contains specific response teams with individual mission focus including

- DMAT—Disaster Medical Assistance Team

- DMORT—Disaster Mortuary Response Team

- NVRT—National Veterinary Response Team

---

[a] The views expressed in this article are those of the author and do not reflect the position or contracted work provided by Battelle Memorial Institute.

National Incident Management System (NIMS). Evaluators also receive additional training on the integrated process and evaluation (IPE) system prior to being part of an exercise. All participants receive a written summary of their performance with strengths, observations, and findings noted.

THE HOSPITAL PREPAREDNESS PROGRAM: CURRENT STATUS

Federal funding for hospitals and the start of the US Hospital Preparedness Program (HPP) began by the passage of the Public Health Security and Bioterrorism Preparedness and Response Act of 2002 and was administered by the US Health Resources and Services Administration (HRSA)[8] of DHHS. The grant program supported health-related activities to prepare for and respond effectively to bioterrorism and other public health emergencies, including the preparation of an emergency preparedness plan. Programmatic emphasis moved to an all-hazards capability-based approach in 2004, and encouraged collaboration in the development of a hazard vulnerability analysis (HVA). The HVA is the base or identification of potential threats to the hospital (or the community), from which all emergency preparedness planning is derived. The HVA is to an emergency preparedness plan as a comprehensive patient history is to developing the nursing care plan; it is difficult to have one without the other if one wants to achieve success.

The Pandemic and All Hazards Preparedness Act of 2006 (PAHPA) created the Office of the Assistant Secretary for Preparedness and Response (ASPR) as the principle advisor to the secretary for DHHS.[9] The HPP program was transferred from HRSA to ASPR, which placed the program in alignment with federal response programs such as NDMS.[10] Within the HPP, the overarching goals include improving medical surge and hospital preparedness. Specific programmatic goals included several items:

- Establishing and maintaining electronic systems to track available hospital beds and other resources through the US National Hospital Available Beds for Emergencies and Disasters (HAvBED) system
- Establishing and maintaining the US Emergency System for Advance Registration of Volunteer Health Professionals (ESAR-VHP) networks—which consist of electronic systems to register, track, and verify the credentials of volunteer health care providers to assist with medical surge during public health emergencies
- Developing health care coalitions and partnerships—networks of health care facilities that can provide medical services, resources, or support during a public health emergency
- Educating and training health care workers
- Implementing and maintaining NIMS activities
- Engaging with other responders through interoperable communications system
- Establishing, maintaining, or enhancing medical countermeasure caches to protect health care workers during an emergency
- Enhancing mass fatality management and evacuation and shelter-in-place plan
- Exercising and improving awardee preparedness plans and coordinating regional exercises

Alignment of the HPP with the US Public Health Emergency Preparedness (PHEP) program occurred in 2012, integrating hospital and public health preparedness and elimination of duplicate goals.[11] The goal of PHEP, which is administered by the US Centers for Disease Control and Prevention (CDC), is to strengthen state and local public health departments' ability to respond to a variety of public health emergencies. Programmatic goals include

- Developing plans to receive, store, distribute, and dispense medical counter-measures during a public health emergency
- Testing awardees' ability to notify and assemble appropriate response staff during an emergency
- Building laboratory capability for testing and identifying harmful pathogens and reporting results to CDC
- Communicating health, risk, and other information in a timely manner to the public in public health emergencies
- Conducting drills and exercises to test response capabilities and activities
- Completing after action reports and improvement plans to improve response times and activities for future drills, exercises, or real events

The need for additional realignment for both the PHEP and HPP programs was described by the US General Accounting Office (GAO) in its March 2013 report.[12] The report noted that progress had been made with some of the capabilities, but was lacking, especially in the area of hospital evacuation. Hospital and health care facility evacuation became a focal event with the landfall of the 2012 Hurricane Sandy in New York City. Hospitals are required to have evacuation plans as part of accreditation and US Centers for Medicare and Medicaid Services (CMS) regulatory requirements; however, they are rarely if ever fully tested due to patient acuity. Flooding and back-up generator failure led to the unplanned evacuation of several large downtown hospitals including New York University (NYU) Langone and Bellevue Hospital. The New York Downtown Hospital evacuated prior to landfall of the hurricane, as did the Veterans Administration Manhattan Hospital. Established relationships with other hospital systems and other elements that were present in the coalition contributed to the successful evacuation of multiple hospitals.[13]

HOSPITAL PREPAREDNESS: MOVING TOWARD HEALTH CARE RESILIENCY THROUGH COALITIONS

One of the hallmarks of PHEP and HPP has been development of coalitions. Coalitions have existed prior to the development of the HPP. Coalitions developed with the CSEPP program, Metropolitan Medical Response System (MMRS), Metropolitan Strike Teams, and now with the hospital preparedness program. Coalitions are locally or regionally based. Membership within coalitions is defined at the local level (city, county, state, or region). Coalitions have established leaders who have specific roles and responsibilities as well as an organizational framework. Individual organizational support is identified through the development of an MOU or memorandum of agreement. Such agreements articulate roles and responsibilities, identify the process for distribution of funding sources, and facilitate the integration of the preparedness community. For example, some coalitions have used HPP grant dollars to purchase equipment, creating communications networks between facilities and first responder partners. They have purchased caches of supplies and established community-based emergency preparedness exercises. Coalitions exist as a result of established day-to-day relationships within a hospital and between hospitals and public health partners. Relationships develop that include levels of trust, familiarity, and dependability. Coalitions have expanded outside the hospital/public health boundaries to include skilled nursing facilities and long term care facilities, all of which are part of the fabric of health care providers in the community. Many coalitions share training schedules, offer joint educational or preparedness conferences, and act as mentors to other health care partners as they develop emergency preparedness plans for their organizations. In times of emergency, knowing one's coalition partners and how to reach them quickly can help keep health care services intact. The ability to bounce back in the face of disaster is the hallmark of resilience.[14] As of 2016, funding levels for both the HPP and

PHEP program have been cut, forcing hospitals to determine whether participation in regional coalitions, planning efforts, and exercises is still worth their financial support.

ON THE HORIZON: CENTERS FOR MEDICARE AND MEDICAID SERVICES REGULATORY REQUIREMENTS

Health care accreditation organizations such as The Joint Commission (TJC), Det Norske Veritas Germanischer Lloyd (DNV-GL), and Health Facilities Accreditation Program (HFAP) have specific requirements for hospital emergency preparedness. The various accreditation standards include common elements such as development of hospital emergency preparedness plans based on a hazard vulnerability analysis, communication plans (inside and outside the hospital), establishment of a hospital incident command system, maintenance of essential environmental controls (heating/cooling/water/sewage), provision of food for patients and staff, patient/staff tracking, enhanced security, and provision of emergency generator power. Hospitals are also required to test their emergency preparedness plans once a year. The new CMS requirements also include participation in an annual community-based disaster exercise and a table-top exercise. Table-top exercises are useful for evaluating specific disaster processes or procedures however, cannot evaluate an emergency preparedness program.

On December 27, 2013, DHHS and CMS issued proposed regulations that build on the many of the existing hospital accreditation standards but also extended preparedness requirements to 17 other entities, including skilled nursing facilities, long-term care, group homes, dialysis facilities, and out patient surgery.[15] Some of the elements contained in the proposed regulations differ from accreditation requirements, specifically with emergency generator testing and the acceptable use of a table-top exercise to test the emergency preparedness plan. CMS released the final rule "Emergency Preparedness Requirements for Medicare and Medicaid Participating Providers and Suppliers" (CMS 3178-F) on September 8, 2016. The regulation goes into effect November 16, 2016 and implementation/compliance is required by November 16, 2017.

SUMMARY

Hospital emergency preparedness is not a new concept, but one that has grown in complexity and importance. Relationships that have developed with other health care partners are important to nurture and contribute to community resilience. Health care coalitions, which include health care partners at every level, are an important part of this process. Federal support for the hospital preparedness program has contributed to greater levels of preparedness for emergencies, both large and small.[16] The nation's communities have come to expect that the health care services they use on a daily basis will be there in the future, even if a disaster occurs.

REFERENCES

1. Scott LA, Ross AP, Schnellmann JF, et al. Surge capability: CHPTER and SC healthcare worker preparedness. J S C Med Assoc 2005;107:74–7.
2. Waugh WL, Streib G. Collaboration and leadership for effective emergency management. Publ Admin Rev 2006;132–40 [Special Issue].
3. Oregon State Civil Defense Council. Annual civil defense report. Portland (OR): Government Printing Office; 1956.
4. Burkle FM, Williams A, Kissoon N. Pediatric emergency mass critical care: the role of community preparedness in conserving critical care resources. Pediatr Crit Care Med 2011;12(Suppl 6):S141–51.

5. Combating terrorism. Observations on the Nunn-Lugar-Domenici Domestic Preparedness Program. 1998. Available at: www.gao.gov/archive/1999/ns99016t.pdf. Accessed March 16, 2016.

6. Destruction of existing stockpile of lethal chemical agents and munitions PL 99–145 Title 14 (B)§1412 -1983. Available at: https://www.gpo.gov/fdsys/pkg/USCODE-2011-title50/pdf/USCODE-2011-title50-chap32-sec1521.pdf. Accessed March 19, 2016.

7. Chemical Stockpile Emergency Preparedness Program. Guidance December 2012. Available at: http://www.fema.gov/media-library-data/20130726-1903-25045-3905/csepp_program_guidance_december_2012.pdf. Accessed March 5, 2016.

8. Public Law 107-188- June 12, 2002. Public Health Security and Bioterrorism Preparedness and response Act of 2002. Available at: https://www.gpo.gov/fdsys/pkg/PLAW-107publ188/pdf/PLAW-107publ188.pdf. Accessed March 5, 2016.

9. The Pandemic and All Hazards Preparedness Act. Available at: https://www.gpo.gov/fdsys/pkg/PLAW-109publ417/pdf/PLAW-109publ417.pdf. Accessed March 5, 2016.

10. The National Disaster Medical System. Available at: http://www.phe.gov/Preparedness/responders/ndms/Pages/default.aspx. Accessed April 12, 2016.

11. CDC-RFA-TP12-1201 Hospital Preparedness Program (HPP) and Public Health Emergency Preparedness (PHEP) cooperative agreements. 2012. Available at: http://www.cdc.gov/phpr/documents/cdc-rfa-tp12-1201_4_17_12_final.pdf. Accessed March 5, 2016.

12. National Preparedness. Improvements needed for measuring awardee performance in meeting medical and public health preparedness and goals. U.S. Government Accountability Office; 2013. Available at: www.gao.gov/assets/66/653259.pdf. Accessed March 5, 2016.

13. Adalja AI, Watson M, Bouri N, et al. Absorbing citywide patient surge during hurricane sandy: a case study in accommodating multiple hospital evacuations. Ann Emerg Med 2014;64(1):66–73.

14. Rambhia K, Waldhorn R, Selck F, et al. A survey of hospitals to determine the prevalence and characteristics of healthcare coalitions for emergency preparedness and response. Biosecur Bioterror 2012;10(3):304–13.

15. Department of Health and Human Services. Centers for Medicare & Medicaid Services. Medicare and Medicaid Programs; emergency preparedness requirements for Medicare and Medicaid Participating Providers and Suppliers; Proposed Rule. 2013. Available at: https://www.gpo.gov/fdsys/pkg/FR-2013-12-27/pdf/2013-30661.pdf. Accessed March 5, 2016.

16. Toner ES, Ravi S, Adalja A, et al. Doing good by playing well with others: Exploring local collaboration for emergency preparedness and response. Health Secur 2015;13(3):281–9.

National Disaster Health Consortium

Competency-Based Training and a Report on the American Nurses Credentialing Center Disaster Certification Development

Sherrill J. Smith, RN, PhD, CNL, CNE*, Sharon L. Farra, RN, PhD, CNE

KEYWORDS

- Disaster education • Competency-based education • Certification
- Interprofessional education • Nursing education

KEY POINTS

- Nurses must be competent in disaster response.
- Education is needed to achieve nurse competencies.
- Interprofessional training facilitates competent practice.
- Certification is a method of validating competency.
- Overcoming barriers is crucial to disaster competency success.

INTRODUCTION

In 2003 the American Nurses Association identified protection of the public as the primary purpose for ensuring the competence of nurses.[1] Competence has been described as professional performance at an expected level. The integration of (1) knowledge, (2) skills, and (3) performance to achieve the expected level of performance is a competency. When individuals display competence they perform at the expected level.[2] Competent practice is needed for disaster response. Disasters are complex events with inherent risks of mortality and morbidity and thus demand specific knowledge and skills. These events require highly trained personnel.

Disclosure: The authors have no commercial or financial conflicts of interest to disclose. The work of the National Disaster Health Consortium has been supported by a grant from Association of Community Health Nurse Educators (Dr S.L. Farra) and the generous support of an anonymous College of Nursing and Health donor.

College of Nursing and Health, Wright State University, 3640 Colonel Glenn Highway, Dayton, OH 45435, USA

* Corresponding author.

E-mail address: sherrill.smith@wright.edu

http://dx.doi.org/10.1016/j.cnur.2016.07.008
0029-6465/16/© 2016 Elsevier Inc. All rights reserved.
nursing.theclinics.com

Disasters are multifaceted events that may be manmade or natural. Most definitions of disaster recognize the need for a response that exceeds current local capability. By their nature, disasters are complicated and often require intervention from interprofessional teams.[3] The response to an emergent event is dependent on the disaster stage and varies depending on the type of incident.[4] To prepare for these events, the World Health Organization[5] has identified as one of its priorities, "Emergency preparedness for effective health response and recovery at all levels. Emergency preparedness, including response planning, training, prepositioning of health supplies, development of surge capacity, and exercises for health care professionals and other emergency service personnel, is critical for the effective performance of the health sector in the response."

Disaster-Specific Competencies

There has been ongoing discussion and development of competencies related to disaster response performance. A multitude of competencies have been identified for health care workers related to disaster preparation, response, and recovery. Some identified competencies include interprofessional; discipline specific, including nursing; specialized professional; and agency specific. Most recently, in response to a call to action to systematically review and improve the discipline of disaster nursing, subject matter experts met to develop the future of disaster nursing, including recommendations for nursing practice, education, policy, and research. From that meeting a recommendation emerged to develop a national set of disaster nursing competencies to be integrated into both American Association of Colleges of Nursing education essentials and the National League for Nursing (NLN) guidelines.[6]

Seminal work related to interprofessional competencies began in 2007 at the direction of the American Medical Association, which brought together experts to develop education competencies for disaster medicine and public health.[7] Building on this framework, an interprofessional group worked to define interprofessional competencies needed by health care professionals to respond to disasters. The result of their work is a structure that presents a method of organizing the diverse competencies into a hierarchical framework.[7] Basic competencies for all health care professions is the basis for the framework, which is depicted in a pyramid design. Progressing up the pyramid, increasingly specific role and discipline competencies are defined (**Fig. 1**).

Nursing Competencies

Disaster-specific competencies for nurses were first described in 2002 by Gebbie and Qureshi,[8] who started the discussion off by identifying core competencies for nurses responding to disasters. Drawing from the public health competencies developed by Gebbie and Qureshi, the team developed the first core competencies for nurses. In 2003, the International Nursing Coalition for Mass Casualty Education (INCME) identified "Educational Competencies for Registered Nurses Responding to Mass Casualty Incidents."[9] The INCME has developed competencies for all nurses as well as materials for meeting those competencies.

Speciality competencies
Within the literature, there are numerous examples of disaster competencies for specific practice areas in nursing. Jorgenson and colleagues[10] describe core competencies for perinatal and neonatal nurses. These competencies correspond to the unique needs of these vulnerable populations by describing measurable objectives addressing the learning needs of nurses caring for these clients. Another exemplar

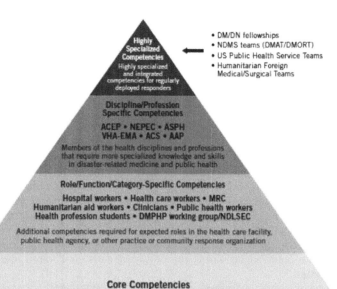

Fig. 1. Hierarchical learning framework. AAP, American Academy of Pediatrics; ACEP, American College of Emergency Physicians; ACS, American College of Surgeons; AMA, American Medical Association; ASPH, Association of Schools of Public Health; CPHPDR, Center for Public Health Preparedness and Disaster Response; DM, Disaster Medicine; DMAT, Disaster Medical Assistance Team; DMORT, Disaster Mortuary Operational Response Team; DMPH, Disaster Medicine and Public Health; DN, Disaster Nursing; ESF-8, Emergency Support Function - #8; EWG, Expert Working Group; FETIG, Federal Education and Training Interagency Group; HSPD-21, Homeland Security Presidential Directive-21; ITS, Integrated Medical, Public Health, Preparedness, and Response Training Summit; KSA, Knowledge, Skills, and Attitudes; MRC, Medical Reserve Corps; NCDMPH, National Center for Disaster Medicine and Public Health; NDLSEC, National Disaster Life Support Education Consortium; NDMS, National Disaster Medical System; NEPEC, Nursing Emergency Preparedness Education Coalition; PAHPA, Pandemic and All-Hazards Preparedness Act; PHP, Public Health Preparedness Summit; TIIDE, Terrorism Injuries: Information Dissemination and Exchange; USUHS, Uniformed Services University of the Health Sciences; VHA-EMA, Veterans Health Administration-Emergency Management Academy. (*Data from* Walsh L, Subbarao I, Gebbie K, et al. Core competencies for disaster medicine and public health. Disaster Med Public Health Prep 2012;6:46; Copyright: Society for Disaster and Public Health.)

of specialty competencies are mental health disaster response competencies. King and colleagues[11] examined competencies developed to guide health professionals in providing mental health care during disasters as a basis for developing effective training programs.

Agency competencies
Other competencies are developed for specific clinical settings. Disaster preparation and response depend on the clinical agency, including type of population served, physical structure, and/or location. For example, Schulz and colleagues[12] have developed national standardized disaster competencies for acute care physicians, nurses, and emergency medical personnel. The competencies and related performance objectives address the specific knowledge, skills, and attitudes required for emergency

department personnel and prehospital emergency care providers. School nursing preparedness needs were described by Mosca and colleagues[13] with an emphasis on bioterrorism response.

As demonstrated by this brief review of competencies, there is great diversity in the expertise and knowledge required by discipline, role, and specific type or location of response. See **Table 1** for a description of these competencies for nursing and nursing specialties over time.

Education and Training to Meet Competencies

Having agreed on standardized competencies is the first step toward developing a disaster-ready nursing workforce; the next logical step is to provide competency-based educational programs with a standardized curricula and performance outcomes.[3,6] It is only through education and training that nurses across the globe can be equipped with the competencies required for responding to disasters.[14] Training and preparation for disasters is not a new endeavor. Education and training opportunities have been developed that include brief self-guided tutorials, day-long field exercises, computer-based virtual reality experiences, and more in-depth graduate level degrees.[4]

In terms of nursing education, a review of the literature noted that no single type of pedagogical approach is superior to any other and that an eclectic approach based on educational objectives aligned with specific disaster competencies is recommended.[15] To date, most disaster education has been provided to practicing health care professionals and most often limited to training targeted at individual specialties.[16] In addition, most educational programs have only been offered in response to a specific event and not based on evidence.[6] Yet, it is recommended that training in disaster competencies occur through interdisciplinary, standardized, competency-based education programs.[4,7] Response to disasters is not limited to one health care specialty; response requires the work of an interprofessional team, including nurses. Interprofessional education has been defined as follows:

> *Interprofessional education occurs when students from two or more professions learn about, from, and with each other to enable effective collaboration and improve health outcomes. Once students understand how to work interprofessionally, they are ready to enter the workplace as a member of the collaborative practice team. This is a key step in moving health systems from fragmentation to a position of strength.[17]*

The goals of interprofessional education are to provide deliberate opportunities for participants to work together to learn to improve individual and community-based outcomes. Based on the Interprofessional Education Collaborative Expert Panel,[18] all professional competencies can be characterized by 3 intersecting types of competencies—individual, unique competencies; shared common competencies; and interprofessional competencies. To develop interprofessional competencies, training must occur in teams of interprofessional providers as they collaborate to provide care that meets individual and population-specific needs.

Exemplar—National Disaster Health Consortium

Based on identified competencies of the hierarchical learning framework, described previously (see **Fig. 1**), an interprofessional competency-based education program was developed—the National Disaster Health Consortium (NDHC). The NDHC program provides health care providers an opportunity to acquire not only basic disaster skill competencies but also opportunities to train and develop interprofessional

Table 1
Nursing disaster competency examples

Gebbie & Qureshi,[8] 2002	Emergency and disaster preparedness: core competencies for nurses	Core competencies 1. Describe the agency's role in responding to a range of emergencies that might arise. 2. Describe the chain of command in emergency response. 3. Identify and locate the agency's emergency response plan. 4. Describe emergency response functions or roles and demonstrate them in regularly performed drills. 5. Demonstrate the use of equipment and the skills required in emergency response during regular drills. 6. Demonstrate the correct operation of all equipment used for emergency communication. 7. Describe communication roles in emergency response. 8. Identify the limits of own knowledge, skills, and authority, and identify key systems resources for referring matters that exceed these limits. 9. Apply creative problem-solving skills and flexible thinking to the situation, within the confines of your role, and EVALUATE the effectiveness of all actions taken. 10. Recognize deviations from the norm that might indicate an emergency and describe appropriate action. 11. Participate in continuing education to maintain up-to-date knowledge in relevant areas. 12. Participate in evaluating every drill or response and IDENTIFY necessary changes to the plan. Leadership competencies 1. Ensure a written plan for major categories of emergencies. 2. Ensure that all parts of the emergency plan are practiced regularly. 3. Ensure that identified gaps in knowledge and skills are filled.
INCME,[9] 2003	Educational competencies for registered nurses responding to mass casualty incidents	Core competencies: critical thinking, assessment (general and specific), technical skills, communication Core knowledge: health promotion, risk reduction, and disease prevention; health care systems and policy; illness and disease management; information and health care technologies; ethics; and human diversity. Professional role development

(continued on next page)

Table 1 (*continued*)		
Mosca and colleagues,[13] 2005	Bioterrorism and disaster training needs of school nurses	9 Bioterrorism and disaster competencies 1. Describe role in emergency response. 2. Describe the chain of command in emergency response. 3. Identify agency emergency response plan. 4. Describe functional roles and demonstrate in drills. 5. Demonstrate correct use of communication equipment. 6. Describe communication roles. 7. Identify limits to knowledge, skills, and authority. 8. Recognize events that would indicate an emergency. 9. Apply creative problem-solving in within functional responsibilities and evaluate effectiveness of actions.
Jorgensen and colleagues,[10] 2010	Emergency preparedness and disaster response core competency set for perinatal and neonatal nurses	Core competency domains 1. Preparation and planning 2. Detection and communication 3. Incident management and support systems 4. Safety and security 5. Clinical and public health assessment and intervention 6. Contingency, continuity, and recovery 7. Public health law and ethics
Schultz and colleagues,[12] 2012	All-hazard disaster core competencies for acute care medical professionals: Emergency department nurses and physicians and out-of-hospital emergency medical services	19 Domains (19 competencies and 90 performance objectives) 1. Nomenclature 2. Incident management systems 3. Recognition, notification, initiation, and data collection 4. Communication (inter/intra-agency, media) 5. Resource management 6. Volunteer management 7. GO-NGO–sponsored response teams 8. Public health safety 9. Patient triage 10. Surge capacity/capability 11. Patient identification and tracking 12. Transportation 13. Decontamination 14. Clinical considerations 15. Special-needs populations 16. Evacuation 17. Critical thinking/situational awareness 18. Ethical principles and challenges 19. Psychosocial issues

(*continued on next page*)

Table 1 (*continued*)		
King and colleagues,[11] 2015	Competencies for disaster mental health in current literature	Mental health competencies 1. Knowledge of the psychological sequelae of disasters 2. Ability to assess and manage mental health issues 3. Ability of responders as caregivers to attend to their own mental health needs 4. General public health professionals competencies: focus on family concerns, such as bereavement, and community-level concerns, such as risk communication and the promotion of community resilience

competencies related to disaster preparation and response. The NDHC training program targets those individuals who may be called on in a disaster but not necessarily working in a disaster management role on a day-to-day basis, including nurses, social workers, pharmacists, physicians, mental health professionals, allied health professionals, health care managers, and first responders in both military and civilian settings.

The NDHC curriculum provides a standardized training program that crosses all phases of the disaster management cycle, including preparedness, response, and recovery, to prepare individuals to work together to develop interprofessional competencies. The hybrid training approach is based on evidence that no one pedagogy may be appropriate but engages participants through reading assignments, online tutorials and discussion opportunities, and an intensive, 4-day on-site immersion with a culminating team-based exercise component emphasizing decision making, leadership, and recovery. The NDHC curriculum is designed to assure that interprofessional, competency-based training pulls all health professionals into compatible training, taking the health care community a significant step closer to a nationwide standardized response to disasters. See **Table 2** for identification of selected competencies, content, and educational delivery method of the NDHC program.

The NDHC competency-based curriculum is divided into components that include prerequisite requirements, online course requirements, and a culminating 4-day intensive experience. Participants have the option of completing coursework for undergraduate/graduate credit or continuing education credit. Prior to taking part in the course, prerequisite activities include completion of 2 Federal Emergency Management Agency (FEMA) courses (IS-100.HCB: Introduction to the Incident Command System [ICS] for Healthcare/Hospitals and IS-200.HCA: Applying ICS to Healthcare Organizations) as well as the National Disaster Life Support Basic Disaster Life Support (BDLS) course. Students are then enrolled into the course learning management system to complete 12 online modules that include unfolding case studies, responding to reading assignments in an online discussion forum, and knowledge assessments using multiple choice quizzes. The program also includes a 4-day, on-site culminating activity that incorporates disaster response scenarios and live exercises in which performance is evaluated using evaluators and exercise-specific performance rating rubrics.

Unique to the NDHC training is the site used for the 4-day final culminating experience. The National Center for Medical Readiness (NCMR) offers a disaster-specific training and research facility located on 54 acres in the city of Fairborn, Ohio. The NCMR training complex, referred to as Calamityville, offers the capability to provide state-of-the art classroom experiences as well as a computer laboratory that serves

Table 2
Summary of National Disaster Health Consortium Training Methods based on competencies

Competency	Educational Content/Delivery
Demonstrate personal and family preparedness for disasters and public health emergencies	Module 1: Disaster defined: History of Disaster: Frameworks and Personal Preparedness (online course module, discussion board, and quiz)
Demonstrate knowledge of one's expected role(s) in organizational and community response plans activated during a disaster or public health emergency.	IS-100.HCB: Introduction to the ICS for Healthcare/Hospitals (online module FEMA). IS-200.HCA: Applying ICS to Healthcare Organizations (online module FEMA). Module 2: Leadership and Coordination in Disaster Health Care Systems (on-site course, discussion board, and quiz)
Demonstrate situational awareness of actual/potential health hazards before, during, and after a disaster or public health emergency.	BDLS course (3.2). Module 2 and Module 2A (face-to-face training with case scenarios)
Communicate effectively with others in a disaster or public health emergency.	Modules 7 and 8: Crisis Leadership Module 9: Crisis Communication/Information Technology in Disaster (on-site modules, discussion boards, and quiz) Community Health and Emergency Operations Center (on-site course with lecture, group scenarios, tabletop, and function exercises)
Demonstrate knowledge of personal safety measures that can be implemented in a disaster or public health emergency.	BDLS course (3.2) (face-to-face lecture with case scenarios) Austere conditions (on-site training and demonstrations)
Demonstrate knowledge of surge capacity assets, consistent with one's role in organizational, agency, and/or community response plans.	BDLS (3.2) Lesson 3 Workforce Readiness and Disaster Deployment (face-to-face training with lecture, scenarios) Surge (on-site course with lecture, tabletop scenarios, and tabletop exercise)
Demonstrate knowledge of principles and practices for the clinical management of all ages and populations affected by disasters and public health emergencies, in accordance with professional scope of practice.	BDLS (3.2) (face-to-face training with lecture and scenarios) Module 10: Infectious Disease Emergencies/Medical Countermeasures Dispensing Module 11: Chemical Terrorism and Surveillance Module 12: Radiological Incidents and Emergencies (on-site modules with lecture, discussion board, and quiz) Triage Principles of Disasters (on-site course, lecture, scenarios, and live exercise) Disaster Response and Recovery Skills (on-site course, didactic scenarios, and exercise)
Demonstrate knowledge of public health principles and practices for the management of all ages and population affected by disasters and public health emergencies.	Module 3: Emergency Health Services and Human Services in Disasters Module 14: Restoring Public Health (on-site modules with lecture, discussion boards, and quizzes) Triage Principles of Disasters (on-site course, lecture, scenarios, and live exercise) Disaster Response and Recovery Skills (on-site course, didactic scenarios, and exercise)

(continued on next page)

Table 2 *(continued)*	
Competency	**Educational Content/Delivery**
Demonstrate knowledge of ethical principles to protect the health and safety of all ages, populations, and communities affected by a disaster of public health emergency.	Module 6: Vulnerable Populations and Disaster Mental Health (online module with lecture, discussion board, and quiz) Ethical and Legal Principles of Disasters (on-site course with case scenarios) Disaster Response and Recovery Skills (on-site course, didactic scenarios, and exercise)
Demonstrate knowledge of legal principles to protect the health and safety of all ages, populations, and communities affected by a disaster or public health emergency.	Module 6: Vulnerable Populations and Disaster Mental Health (online module with lecture, discussion boards, and quizzes) Ethical and Legal Principles of Disasters (on-site course with lecture and case scenarios)
Demonstrate knowledge of short-term and long-term considerations for recovery of all ages, populations, and communities affected by a disaster or public health emergency.	Module 5: Hospital and Emergency Department Emergency Preparedness Module 6: Vulnerable Populations and Disaster Mental Health Module 14: Restoring Public Health (online modules with lecture, discussion boards, and quizzes)

as an alternate site for the state's Emergency Operations Center. Simulation laboratories, with both high-fidelity and other static models that include extensive moulage options, allow opportunities for both skill training and scenario-based training for disaster. Unique to the setting is a former cement plant structure providing realistic opportunities for search and recovery training and an actual medical transport helicopter for practicing loading/unloading patients for rotary wing transport. The training complex also offers other realistic disaster response opportunities, such as loading patients into a school bus, extrication from motor vehicles, and responding to a residential area after a tornado to enhance the realism of training and preparation for disaster response.[19] See **Figs. 2–4** for pictures of NDHC on-site activities held at the NCMR site.

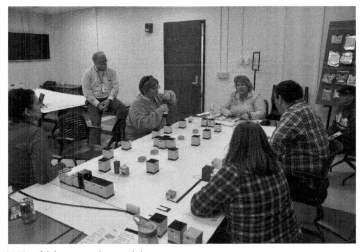

Fig. 2. NDHC vehicle extraction activity.

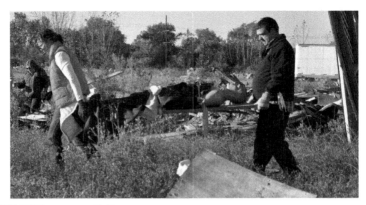

Fig. 3. NDHC litter carry activity.

National Center for Medical Readiness Calamityville Training Complex

In 2014, more than 50 acres of land in Fairborn, Ohio, were transferred from the city of Fairborn to Wright State University, for the NCMR Calamityville disaster training complex. The site of a former cement plant, the complex underwent several years of cleanup and construction to prepare the site for disaster training activities. The complex includes both classrooms and more than 10 different simulated disaster areas offering training in response to hazardous materials, rescue from confined spaces, and practice of rescue as well as emergency transport using a variety of vehicles. With its close proximity to Wright-Patterson Air Force Base, collaborative training opportunities have been provided to military personnel. Training has been offered to health care personnel as well as school personnel, fire fighters, forensic anthropologists, and funeral directors. Projects have been developed not only with Wright State University departments but also other local research institutes and community colleges. The site has also been used to test and develop state-of-the art technology for disaster

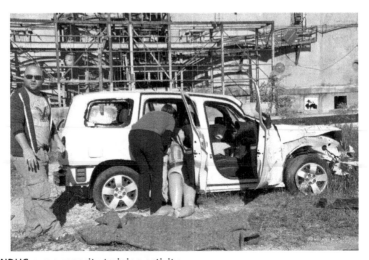

Fig. 4. NDHC surge capacity training activity.

response, such as radiofrequency identification technology capability and combining virtual reality experiences with on-site training.[19–21]

Over the past year, the NDHC training program has been offered 5 times with 136 participants completing the program. Participants have primarily been nurses and nursing faculty; however, other professionals completing the program have been emergency management directors, paramedics, principals and staff from local school districts, military personnel, and Veterans Affairs medical staff. Feedback has primarily been positive, with comments, such as "I enjoyed the opportunity to participate at a facility that is capable of designing an exercise that mocks a disaster scene" and "I learned so much and will retain that information much better since I was able to perform skills." Participants in the program have been able to leave the program to implement disaster-specific content into nursing curricula, develop agency-specific disaster preparedness and policies, and even return to volunteer as instructors in future courses. Specific information about the NDHC courses and outcomes are published elsewhere.[22]

Certification

Nursing and other professionals must demonstrate competency and readiness for entry-level practice, generally conducted through a process of licensure by examination. Licensure, however, does not guarantee competency in specialty areas of practice. The standard for demonstration of competent, evidence-based care in a specialty area of practice is certification. Although early evidence indicated a correlation between positive outcomes and nurse certification, lack of reliable and valid current evidence to demonstrate whether positive outcomes, such as quality patient care and patient satisfaction, are related to certification limits ability to predict impact of professional certification. This lack of evidence suggests a need for examining the structure and processes of certification with combined efforts by both certification accrediting bodies and education partners to develop programs that adequately prepare professionals to gain the specialty knowledge, skills, and attitudes to make a difference in patient outcomes.[23]

In addition, as discussed previously, regarding disaster education, certification for disaster specialty cannot ignore the importance of the interprofessional nature of disaster care. Nurses do not care for patients in a multicasualty event or disaster in isolation of providers from a variety of specialties. A needs analysis conducted to determine the potential market for a disaster certificate program for nurses and other health care professionals noted a gap that could be filled with a hybrid educational program preparing health care providers for disaster certification. This analysis, conducted in 2012, examined labor market trends both nationally and regionally in terms of disaster preparedness, especially in terms of health care professions. In addition, the analysis included an examination of the potential demand for both generic disaster training and training specific to health care personnel. Finally, an examination of current training opportunities was conducted. Based on the analysis, recommendations for a hybrid disaster certificate program with proposed outcomes was identified.[24] This training model led to collaboration with the American Nurses Credentialing Center to develop the National Healthcare Disaster Certification specialty certification. This new certification currently is in the development phase and acknowledges the interprofessional nature of disaster and need for not just a nursing specialty certification but one that demonstrates the interprofessional competencies required for disaster care. As with other certifications, the National Healthcare Disaster Certification will provide employers and the public overall the assurance of interprofessional disaster-specific competencies across all aspects of the disaster cycle.[25]

DISCUSSION

The need for competency-based education and recognition of competency through certification is clear and most likely without argument. The NDHC hopes to assist in preparing health professionals with the knowledge, skills, and attitudes needed for certification. The next step in having competent practitioners is to ensure health care professionals are prepared when disaster strikes through access to training opportunities and preparation for meeting disaster certification competencies. Since the Institute of Medicine *The Future of Nursing* report published in 2010, recommendations to improve nursing care through initiatives, such as collaborative educational models, have been offered and such collaborations are still needed to meet the complex health care needs of individual patients and communities.[26] Disasters are one of the most complex health care situations any provider might encounter. Nurses encompass the largest group of health care providers and providing nurses access to training opportunities is one step toward meeting goals of promoting individual patient and community-based client needs as well as protecting the safety of nurses. This training must be competency based and provide opportunities to demonstrate abilities required for nursing specifically across levels, such as competencies integrated into American Association of Colleges of Nursing and NLN educational competencies.[6]

Training must also include, however, opportunities for all health care professionals and identifying actual interprofessional health care teams to train and learn together to enhance outcomes after an actual disaster. To make this happen, barriers must be identified and addressed. Barriers to implementation of disaster education and competency development include individual, organizational, and environmental barriers.[6] Barriers to the NDHC-specific implementation include the cost and time commitment required for training. The current monetary cost for training has been a significant barrier to many professionals; this barrier is being addressed by soliciting grants for scholarships for individuals to pay for the cost of the training. The scholarships, however, do not cover travel or lodging expenses that also are required for anyone to travel to this unique setting because access to similar training is not yet universally available across the country. Another barrier is the required time commitment. All working health professionals must juggle the demands of professional and personal expectations; disaster competencies are only one competency required for safe practice. Although the online component is designed in a way to allow participants to engage in the material without a synchronicity requirement, the NDHC time commitments of prerequisites and online requirements are lengthy. The culminating 4-day experience requiring time away from work is especially challenging. Many providers may not be able to obtain time off with pay or do not have the available vacation days to be away from their employment to be able to participate. When actual work teams were asked to participate for this amount of time, the need to cover for a large number of employees for almost an entire week was burdensome and difficult for health care settings to manage. These barriers must be addressed to be able to ensure feasibility and long-term sustainability of such a training endeavor.

SUMMARY

Meeting the need to prepare and respond to disasters across the globe is complex. Although disaster competencies have been developed, health care providers must be able to respond with unique individual professional disaster competencies as well as those required to work in interprofessional teams. Having standardized training programs, like the NDHC, paves the way for standardizing training to meet competencies with an eclectic, adult-focused format that also provides the background needed for competency documented through certification. Barriers to education and training must first be addressed as well as creation of interdisciplinary opportunities to have the available competent health care providers to respond to protect both individuals and communities in the future whenever disaster strikes.

ACKNOWLEDGMENTS

The authors thank Jack Smith, Jim Gruenberg, and Daniel Kirkpatrick for their contributions in the conception and development of the National Disaster Health Consortium program and Kelly Hanlon for her assistance with the development of this article.

REFERENCES

1. American Nurses Association. Definition of nursing. 2003. Available at: http://www.nursingworld.org/FunctionalMenuCategories/FAQs. Accessed March 15, 2016.
2. American Nurses Association. DRAFT Position Statement on Competence and Competency. 2007. Available at: http://www.nursingworld.org/DocumentVault/draftCompetenceCompetencyPositionStatement.tx. Accessed March 15, 2016.
3. Ripoll Gallardo A, Djalali A, Foletti M, et al. Core competencies in disaste rmanagement and humanitarian assistance: a systematic review. Disaster Med Public Health Prep 2015;9(4):430–9.
4. Stanley SAR, Wolanski TAB. Designing and integrating a disaster preparedness curriculum: readying nurses for the worst. Indianapolis (IN): Sigma Theta Tau International; 2015.
5. World Health Organization (WHO). Emergency risk management for health overview. The United Nations Office for disaster risk Reduction. Geneva (Switzerland): World Health Organization (WHO); 2013. Available at: http://www.who.int/hac/techguidance/preparedness/risk_management_overview_17may2013.pdf?ua=1.
6. Veeenema TG, Griffin A, Gable AR, et al. Nurses as leaders in disaster preparedness and response-A Call to action. J Nurs Scholarsh 2016;48(2):187–200.
7. Walsh L, Subbarao I, Gebbie K, et al. Core competencies for disaster medicine and public health. Disaster Med Public Health Prep 2012;6:44–52.
8. Gebbie K, Qureshi K. Emergency and disaster preparedness: Core competencies for nurses. Am J Nurs 2002;102(1):46–51.
9. International Nursing Coalition for Mass Casualty Education (INCME). Educational competencies for registered nurses responding to mass casualty incidents. 2003. Available at: http://www.aacn.nche.edu/leading-initiatives/education-resources/INCMCECompetencies.pdf. Accessed March 15, 2016.
10. Jorgensen AM, Mendoza GJ, Henderson JL. Emergency preparedness and disaster response core competency set for perinatal and neonatal nurses. J Obstet Gynecol Neonatal Nurs 2010;39(4):450–65.
11. King RV, Burkle FM Jr, Walsh LE, et al. Competencies for disaster mental health. Curr Psychiatry Rep 2015;17(3):548.
12. Schultz CH, Koenig KL, Whiteside M, et al. Development of national standardized all-hazard disaster core competencies for acute care physicians, nurses, and EMS professionals. Ann Emerg Med 2012;59(3):196–208.
13. Mosca NW, Sweeney PM, Hazy JM, et al. Assessing bioterrorism and disaster preparedness training needs for school nurses. J Public Health Manag Pract 2005;(Suppl):S38–44.

14. Weiner E. Preparing nurses internationally for emergency planning and response. Online J Issues Nurs 2006;11(3):4.

15. Jose M, Dufrene C. Educational competencies and technologies for disaster preparedness in undergraduate nursing education: An integrative review. Nurse Educ Today 2014;34:543–51.

16. Miller JL, Rambeck JH, Snyder A. Improving emergency preparedness system readiness through simulation and interprofessional education. Public Health Rep 2014;129(4):129–35.

17. World Health Organization (WHO). Framework for action on interprofessional education and collaborative practice. Geneva (Switzerland): World Health Organization (WHO); 2010. Available at: http://whqlibdoc.who.int/hq/2010/WHO_HRH_HPN_10.3_eng.pdf.

18. Interprofessional Education Collaborative Expert Panel. Core competencies for interprofessional collaborative practice. Washington, DC: Interprofessional Education Collaborative; 2011. Available at: https://ipecollaborative.org/uploads/IPEC-Core-Competencies.pdf.

19. National Center for Medical Readiness (NCMR). National center for medical readiness website. Wright State University; 2016. Available at: https://www.wright.edu/national-center-for-medical-readiness.

20. Mathews S. Wright State to take over Calamityville property. Dayton Daily News 2014. Available at: http://www.mydaytondailynews.com/news/news/local-govt-politics/wright-state-to-take-over-calamityville-property/nhyGP/?icmp=daytondaily_internallink_textlink_apr2013_daytondailystubtomydaytondaily_launch.

21. Hannah J. Wright State University taking ownership of Calamityville. 2014. Available at: https://webapp2.wright.edu/web1/newsroom/2014/11/03/wright-state-university-takes-ownership-of-calamityville/. Accessed March 15, 2016.

22. Farra S, Smith S, Bashaw M. Learning outcome measurement in nurse participants following disaster training. Disaster Med Public Health Prep 2016;1–6.

23. Martin LC, Arenas-Montoya NM, Barnett TO. Impact of nurse certification rates on patient satisfaction and outcomes: a literature review. J Contin Educ Nurs 2015; 46(12):549–54.

24. Hanover Research. Disaster preparedness certificate program program demand prepared for Wright State University. Washington, DC: Hanover Research; 2012.

25. American Nurses Credentialing Center. National Healthcare Disaster Certification. 2016. Available at: http://www.nursecredentialing.org/Certification/DisasterCertification. Accessed March 15, 2016.

26. Institute of Medicine. Assessing progress on the institute of medicine report the future of nursing. Washington, DC: The National Academies Press; 2015. Available at: http://iom.nationalacademies.org/Reports/2015/Assessing-Progress-on-the-IOM-Report-The-Future-of-Nursing.aspx.

All the Resources was Gone
The Environmental Context of Disaster Nursing

Stasia E. Ruskie, PhD, RN

KEYWORDS

- Disaster • Nursing • Disaster environment • Infrastructure • Preparedness

KEY POINTS

- The health care sector depends on an enabling societal infrastructure of support systems, including power, water, and communications.
- In a disaster setting, these infrastructural resources may only minimally function.
- Reduced infrastructure resources in disaster environments impacts US nurses' capability and their physical and emotional health.
- Nursing education, practice, training, and research should integrate disaster health care preparedness with the likely disaster conditions of providing that health care.

BACKGROUND

Much of US nurses' disaster preparedness training is hospital- and emergency department–based. Nurses routinely participate in disaster triage and decontamination drills involving high-intensity, high-acuity chemical, biologic, radiologic, nuclear, and explosive (CBRNE) mass casualty incidents (MCIs) generally staged in fully functioning, fully resourced health care and community settings. Yet US nurses consistently report their discomfort with the "unexpected," "unfamiliar," and "unusual" circumstances of the disaster environment they encountered while providing emergency health care. Nursing during disaster has been described as "nursing in hell,"[1] and the disaster conditions as "hostile and austere"[2] and worse than those in combat.[3]

In primarily first-person accounts, US nurses have described their "general lack of knowledge" and readiness for the altered conditions and damaged surroundings in the landscape of the disaster environment. They were unprepared for extended work-shifts, overwhelming numbers of patients, the prevalence of medical and chronic illnesses, inadequate amounts of medical supplies and equipment, and the emotional health needs of patients and responders during their disaster responses.[1–4]

Beyond health care, they also described the hardships of extreme temperatures; minimalist sleeping and living conditions; portable, rudimentary, or nonfunctional

Disclosures: None.
1729 Martha Street, NE, Albuquerque, NM 87112, USA
E-mail address: stasia.ruskie@gmail.com

Nurs Clin N Am 51 (2016) 569–584
http://dx.doi.org/10.1016/j.cnur.2016.07.011
0029-6465/16/© 2016 Elsevier Inc. All rights reserved.
nursing.theclinics.com

water, sanitation, electrical, and communications systems; and unfamiliarity with cultural standards and the existence of extreme poverty.[5–8] Feelings of personal incompetence while working in these difficult conditions[1] contributed to nurses' emotionally and physically exhausting disaster experiences.[7–10]

A growing body of research documents the long-term adverse health outcomes, including increased anxiety, altered coping, and posttraumatic stress disorder in disaster workers and health care providers.[11–14] Factors contributing to these ill-effects are not well understood, and focus on nurses' personal attributes.[15,16] More specifically, despite nurses' graphic portrayals of the altered conditions and the reduced resources surrounding nurses during their disaster health care response, the disaster environment has not been included as part of disaster preparedness training, nor has it been a focus of disaster or nursing research.

PURPOSE

This study focuses on the overlooked background context of disaster nursing, and explicitly describes the disaster environment experienced by US nurses during their disaster health care response.

METHOD
Study Design

A qualitative research approach, appropriate for initial discovery when little is known about a phenomenon,[17,18] was used to guide the larger study from which this environmental description of disaster nursing was taken. In the existential phenomenologic philosophy of Merleau-Ponty,[19] the figural aspects that stand out from an experience can only be understood by understanding the context of the world that surrounds and cocreates that experience. This perspective provides a coherent philosophy for examining the context of the disaster nursing environment.

Data Collection

Following institutional review board approval, participants who had participated in a major disaster as a registered civilian nurse were recruited from US national and state nursing associations. Digitally recorded interviews were conducted in person (eight) or via Skype (three). After obtaining informed consent, participants were asked: "When you think about your disaster environment, what stands out about your experience?" Interviews were transcribed verbatim and verified for accuracy. Pseudonyms replaced all potentially identifying information to ensure participant anonymity.

Data Analysis

Data were analyzed followed Thomas and Pollio's[20] methodology based on Merleau-Ponty's existential philosophy. Common experiences of the disaster environment were discerned across all interviews. Study reliability was enhanced via an understanding of the philosophic basis of the chosen phenomenological research method, obtaining data saturation (the point were no new data are being discovered from additional interviews), and through prolonged immersion in the study data.[21–23] Using open-ended questions and encouraging participants to speak freely about their disaster experience provided internal validity, or the credibility of the data itself.[21,22] Participants' abundant details of their experiences, the use of their own words to support all study conclusions, and the concurrence of study conclusions by participants (member checking)[21,22,24] further support the analytical rigor of this study.

RESULTS

At the time of their interviews, participants (10 women, one male) resided in seven states and one foreign country. With an average age of 57, they had a mean of 25.9 years nursing experience. Nurses had widely varied specializations, and 82% held an advanced nursing degree. Nurses had participated in 1 to more than 25 disaster events, primarily in the United States, including hurricanes, derechos (high-intensity straight-line winds with thunderstorms), flooding, tornados, bombings, earthquakes, train derailments, water system contaminations, and communicable disease outbreaks. Their experiences lasted from one 8-hour shift to more than 180 days. Their self-described disaster training included "none," "general hospital preparedness training," specialized certifications, specific emergency and disaster training, and master's degrees (see participant demographics in **Table 1**). Three nurses worked fulltime in disaster response; one as a high level administrator. The remaining study nurses had directly experienced a disaster, or deployed as a disaster volunteer.

THE ENVIRONMENT OF DISASTER

Nurses in this study described disaster environments that were "not normal," and where "all the resources" of society "were gone." Working without "staff," "stuff," or "systems," the altered and damaged conditions were "unexpected," not "what we're used to," a "swirling ... mass" of "disorder" where nurses had "no control." The continual non–health care challenges created situations where nurses were unable to follow the usual structure of nursing training, hospital policy, and health care laws and regulations, and the nursing environment became "chaos and... tension and... stress."

Health Care Environment of Disaster

In some disasters, nurses worked in their undamaged, but nevertheless altered, hospital or public health department setting. In many other situations, the nurses' usual worksites were destroyed. Nurses provided health care in numerous unexpected alternate care settings: "the crosstown hospital's overcrowded emergency department," "mass shelters," "make-shift...triage tents," a "civic auditorium," "athletic stadium," or "in the field."

Whether in relative or actual numbers, nurses had too many patients for the altered conditions. In a hospital without power, water, or food during a flood, "once patients could come in, we'd have to transfer 'em out" (RN5). In an alternate care facility "we ... basically triaged sixteen thousand people" (RN4).

Overwhelmed with patients, nurses had insufficient staff or had staff without relevant expertise. An "obstetrics-trained physician" and an "ophthalmologist" were "running" a "cholera treatment center." A physician who "didn't know how to [perform focused disaster] triage" quickly became "overwhelmed" trying to provide detailed hospital assessments for the enormous influx of patients. A volunteer physician responded as if he was located in a fully functional hospital instead of in a civic auditorium overflowing with frightened survivors:

> ...he says, "I need a complete blood count and an electrocardiogram stat," and I'm like, "We've had a tornado. We don't have any lab here. We don't have an electrocardiogram machine yet." ... And he was kind of like, looking at me like, "Well, why not?" You know? [Laughs] I was like, "We had a tornado!" (RN11)

Table 1 Participant characteristics	
Variable	**Number of Nurses**
Ethnicity	
White	10
Hispanic	1
Sex	
Female	10
Male	1
Education	
ADN	1
BSN	1
MSN/MS	6
DNP	2
PhD	1
Nursing specialty	
Medical-surgical	3
Public health	2
Family health	1
Geriatric	1
Pediatrics	3
Forensics	1
Emergency/trauma nursing	4
Cardiovascular	1
Self-defined disaster training	
None	2
General hospital preparedness training	1
Red Cross training	2
Master's degree in disaster preparedness	2
Basic and Advanced Disaster Life Support	1
Hazmat training	2
Trauma Nursing Core Course	2
National Incident Management System Incident Command System courses	4
Federal homeland defense and disaster courses	3
State training	1
Medical Reserve Corps	1
Emergency	1
Public health	1

Nurses could identify multiple specialties, training, so N >11.

Along with insufficient staff, nurses also worked without their accustomed clinical equipment and supplies. Nurses "were kind of by the seat of their pants" (RN2) and had to "make do with what they had" (RN5):

We don't have any more supplies for the physician, we don't have a clean scalpel, we don't have … we're just digging through boxes and we found, of all things, some mint-flavored [rubbing] alcohol. Why in the world we ever had such a thing. And I looked at this operating room nurse and I said, "You know how to sterilize things. Will this work?" She said, "It's all we got," you know, so we used it. ... I mean, you just put together what you had to (RN11).

When responding to their own locally occurring disasters, nurses only described the altered surroundings affecting them and their patients. Nurses who volunteered for distant events named populations of survivors that stood out during their experience. Two of the experienced deploying nurses explained how certain groups in society are more vulnerable to disaster harm. Most nurses who deployed to disasters identified the racial, social, economic, cultural, or health care status of people that stood out to them (**Box 1**). Several explained how the disaster brought together populations that "would not normally interact," because of "socially-created separations." Nurses specifically mentioned "poor," "undocumented," "homeless and the drug addicts," "a whole bunch of group-home schizophrenics," "persons who are pregnant," "a women's group for battered women" co-located in a shelter with the offending men "from the halfway house," "gangs," "black persons," "Vietnamese," and "Spanish/ Mexican" people.

Nurses were also surprised to encounter racial prejudices:

I was a ...white boy going into some of these [southern state] areas that, you know, they didn't want you there. Or, then ... when I was in [midwest state] ... where my partner was a black nurse and they wanted no part of that. So it was having to deal with some of my naive ideas, coming from [northern state], that this stuff is still out there (RN6).

Box 1

Survivor groups described by nurses

RN1: You had families with children that had not evacuated, and they were trying to live in the shelter. And then you've got a drug ... addict that's wanting to steal things, trying to go through people's stuff, ... threatening them if they have any narcotics, you know, "You have cigarettes? You have any alcohol with you?" that kind of thing. ...That was freaking people out, obviously. ... it was not a safe shelter as long as those people were there pursuing their habits.

RN2: There were people ... of all races, of all ages, ... several different ethnic communities, ... persons with disabilities, ... a whole population of people on methadone.

RN3: And, honestly, the populations that you are dealing with in disaster, that I have dealt with in disaster, by and far they're my public health populations. They're already vulnerable. They're already at risk.

RN4: People that have been displaced, you know, a whole nursing home full of patients arrived at this gym.

RN5: (Local) Patient-wise, ... the staff, everybody pretty much knew what to do.

RN6: They had a large black population; you had a Spanish/Mexican population.

RN8: (Local) Their first priority was to take care of anybody that needed to be taken care of.

RN9: If anyone had mental health issues, um, and they were off their medications, they got closer to us... I noticed that people that had families or children – 'cause when you – when you looked down into the concourse, there's all these tents.

RN10: And so, uh, yeah, so you had all these kind of cultural things playing into it as well. And then, like I had some issues with the Haitian staff, who... really were not used to having jobs.

RN11: (Local) What stands out the most is how people from all over who've never met one another came together and did great care for patients.

This "mixing of cultural norms" along with the stress of disaster created a charged atmosphere in shelter settings where "you've taken … ten pounds of flour and put it in a five-pound bag" (RN6).

The Disaster Environment Surrounding Disaster Health Care

The nonexistence of or damage to expected societal infrastructural support systems dramatically affected the care nurses could provide in the disaster environment (**Box 2**). A hurricane evacuation shelter "lost sewer … [and] lost drinking water" for 3 days. A triage tent had "no bathroom" for patients. Public health standards became

---

Box 2
Descriptions of the disaster environment

RN1: There was no electricity to operate the pharmacies, the same situation as with the grocery stores and the gas stations. They didn't have a… computer system where they could see who had what kind of prescription, so they couldn't fill prescriptions unless you could show a bottle that said there was refills on it. … there was no insurance because that's all computer and electronic, too, so you had to be prepared to pay cash money for any medication that you got. And some medicines, if you don't have your insurance, are just through the roof, an impossibility to… purchase them,… unless you got a couple of thousand dollars in cash… around the house, and most people don't.

RN1: [We were housed in] a warehouse with two hundred people… that were mostly male…and that was weird. Plus …. military… troops that were in there too.

RN2: I was horrified at the things that weren't working …communication, strategies, process, things that just did not work very well.

RN3: You think … you've got it all down and it goes to hell in a handbasket, any planning you had made.

RN4: These are things that nobody thought about… all the ramifications if you don't have water in a hospital. … what happens to the surgery or… how are you gonna wash your hands on the unit, how are you gonna flush the toilets.

RN5: You were on minimal staff. And that got tiring after a while.

RN6: These fields would fill up with coiled snakes. …It became a minefield going out to the [shelter] outhouse. … You don't think of those things. And then … all these black widows started showing up.

RN7: It just was … a large open space that would be rented out for… community activities. … Has some …. auditorium seating, but then… a large floor, flat, … open space. …. And…the hospital set up the areas of the hospital. … (demonstrating with hands) here's the neuro floor in this row of tables and here's the … cardiac floor, this row of tables and then, you know, triage was at this end….

RN8: It was chaos … in the environment, …. with the structures of the building… being down, with there being lots of noise, lots of… sirens, lots of… dust, lots of…unsureness of what was going on.

RN9: There were like all of these tents set up … where families lived, and then some people didn't have tents and some people had … those tarps that were set up.

RN10: We had tanks that held feces. … You literally had to go dump buckets of output into containers and, of course, infection control and avoiding cross-contamination was a big deal.

RN11: The generator didn't function, so that's why we did lose, I believe it was, five or six patients… on ventilators and one of 'em was struck by a beam falling and there wouldn't have been anything we could do for that, but the others … were on ventilators. Of course, they quit working. But if that generator had worked, a lot of people would have been electrocuted because there was all kinds of wiring and everything down. And so, really, even though it was bad, it was a blessing that it didn't work.

difficult to maintain. During disaster, the environment was full of "dirt," "debris and stuff," "flies," and "mice" that nurses "would not normally be exposed to."

The communications infrastructure "fell apart." Cell towers were "knocked down" or had limited access because they "had a lot of calls on them." In a shelter, "the telephones didn't work." State-level health department messages "didn't get" to the affected county's health department.

Because of the loss of systems and supplies, nursing became "hands on: sensory, self-reliant, not technology, but personal again" (RN4). Nurses described it as "basic nursing care" and "jungle nursing." They provided food, water, first aid, and emotional support for traumatized and scared survivors, and managing chronic medical conditions exacerbated by the disaster stress (**Box 3**). Because of these altered conditions,

---

Box 3
Descriptions of "basic nursing"

RN1: A lot of people trying to take medication didn't have the right food to go with the, didn't have water to wash it down with. It got tough.

RN2: When it's 94°F and 94% humidity ... to keep that shelter habitable, it had to have air conditioning. ... We needed wool blankets to help people at ... night because ... it was cold in the air conditioning.

RN3: It's population focus. You're looking to fix systems, to put them back into place.... I'm talking about the types of ...nursing care that public health nurses do on that bigger level and ... stringing those systems together, pulling in those resources, ... assessing, assuring, ... developing policy on the fly, if you will, you know, your core functions of public health.

RN4: I would say most of the ... people that we treated, a lot of 'em had chronic medical conditions that were exacerbated because they didn't have their medications. There weren't ventilators and stuff like that. I mean, a lot of people just needed food. They hadn't eaten in several days. Maybe wound care. ... So it was more reassuring people, counseling people. We had mental health professionals that were there...And even for the staff we had ... critical incident stress management offered ... every day.

RN5: The water came so fast that it was very easy ... to have ... some slight injuries, you know, cuts, bruises, so we were going back, checking all those. Making sure people had their medicines, did we need to call somebody to get medicines in and things like that.

RN6: It was basic nursing 101, duct tape and Band-Aids and emotional support, ... spiritual support,... right down to ... the top three physical needs of food, water, shelter.

RN7: The environment was so drastically different than where... we had worked in our nice, plush little hospital and we'd complain when it was a little too hot or a little too cold ... we learned how to make do and take care of the patients the best you can and take care of the needs of the patient with what you've got.

RN8: I was kind of astounded that we were able to function in an outside environment in a field... with very little supplies. ...We had enough to be able to start intravenous lines, we had enough to be able to... bandage ... people up.

RN9: The [organization name] said that ... we were not allowed to dispense any medications.

RN10: If someone came in pulseless and still breathing, we just got fluids into 'em. But there was no point in taking a blood pressure. ... So, yeah, it was kind of crazy, because a lot of my background is the intensive care unit and pediatric cardiac and all this. ...It was a very different kind of environment. So later on, we got ... one heart monitor but we didn't use it very often. We certainly didn't put it on everyone. Later on, we got some oxygen. We had none for the first couple of months.

RN11: A lot of it was using just your eyes and your hands. You know, do I feel a rapid pulse or not? And ... yeah, you ... get some very basic nursing skills back onboard. [Laughs] You don't have a monitor to tell you what's happening.

nurses broke health care rules and policies (**Box 4**) to provide the best care possible under the irregular circumstances.

Physical Effects on Nurses

With the loss of infrastructural capabilities, providing health care became physically demanding for these nurses. "The work conditions were tough. It was such a complete devastation" (RN6). The altered conditions were "freaky" and "scary," and security and safety were a large concern for these nurses. One nurse was told to seek shelter from further threatening weather in her just-destroyed hospital. Nurses labored in climatologic extremes. "It was a 110°F heat index and people were sweaty and gross and they were wearing the clothes that they were wearing before the storm" (RN1).

These altered environmental contexts created "an impossible level of work" for nurses. Clinics, care facilities, and shelters often functioned 24 hours a day. Nurses frequently worked extended shifts with no days off: "16 hours," "20 hours," "26 or 28 hours," or until the work "was done." Previously mechanized health care tasks were accomplished via energy- and time-consuming manual methods. The arduous work shifts, climatologic extremes, and limited rest and recuperation all contributed to nurses being "sleep-deprived," "pretty fatigued," and "exhausted."

Box 4
Breaking rules, regulations, policies, and laws in the disaster setting

RN1: The regulations and the policies that we normally.... follow are set aside.

RN2: The first... disaster was a way of really getting to test what were the things I had been trained on and how did it actually apply in the field and... what did you need to do... differently than what was in the playbook.

RN3: It is being street smart about what you keep and what you kick out the door at that minute in terms of ... what is protocol, what is not, ... and, yes, all that can come back and bite you later if you are not ... doing some good decision-making there. And it's about risk. How much risk ... are you as a practitioner willing to take? How much are you willing to take for yourself while still keeping the clients safe?

RN4: When you have basically your infrastructure gone, the hospitals were overwhelmed. ... I mean, we actually had chest pain patients coming to the athletic center.

RN5: We gave everybody the wrong foods.... "Low salt diet? Oh, here, have a bologna sandwich. Enjoy yourself. That's all we got."

RN6: I stole a telephonebook from a gas station 'cause I'm like, we need resources, ... and I was like, "We gotta find stuff, people."

RN7: We had four by four gauze pads. They were wet, but we had four by four gauze pads.

RN8: You have to use the knowledge that you have... and to process that very quickly,.... to make decisions that normally you wouldn't be making, that... maybe a physician or a resident or an intern... would [normally] be making.

RN9: We were ... getting a bunch of red tape and we couldn't figure out how to [be officially deployed]. So she said, "Well, I'm just gonna go."

RN10: Forget what the hospital tells you, you never changed your intravenous tubing unless...it had a hole in it, because you just didn't have enough.

RN11: We put people in these vehicles with strangers, hoping that they were gonna take 'em over to the other hospital. We didn't know for sure who they were... and you just hope for the best.

Psychosocial Impact on Nurses

Nurses described their "shock" and "disbelief" at the "intense" surroundings of their disaster environment and from seeing "so much need all around." Nurses shed "a lot of tears," "lost it," and were "overwhelmed" with the "stress," the "tension," and the enormity of the suffering. Around them, their colleagues were "psychologically fried," "nonfunctional," or having a "meltdown."

Study participants acknowledged their lingering adverse psychosocial effects. "Even, you know, 10, 15, 20 years after this has happened, it still brings up emotions" (RN8). Another nurse attributed her long-term emotional distress to being immersed in an environment of human and physical devastation:

> Probably all of us should have had some counseling. You know, I wasn't there when the storm went through, but the things I saw, I had nightmares for 29 days, exactly 29 days, every night. ... Thinking back ... that was definitely stress-related. ... I do know of some nurses that ... were not there [during the actual tornado impact] that had some pretty traumatic posttraumatic stress disorder [RN7].

Lack of Preparedness

Study nurses readily admitted their inadequacy for the disaster conditions they encountered (**Box 5**). "I wasn't prepared for where I was going to work. I wasn't prepared for what supplies we had to use" (RN7). Critiquing current disaster preparedness, one nurse expressed:

> I just wanna puke. It is unbelievable to me, having been in the disaster world for 15 years, that we think we bring nurses in and teach them how to extract people from cars and vehicles and ... tell them about the systems we have in place – oh, that's another big one, Here's the systems and they're gonna work for you – until they don't work, which is about the first hour in – and, by the way, here's how you triage your patients, as if that's all there is to learn (RN3).

Nurses in this study were physically and psychologically unprepared for the unexpected and under resourced "not normal" disaster environment conditions. Nursing was a "small piece" of the "multiple challenges" arising from the broader disruption of the disaster environment around them.

DISCUSSION

Current hospital preparedness drills that simulate MCIs, CBRNE, and surge events are in reality addressing medical disaster, or a "catastrophic event that results in casualties that overwhelm the health care resources of the community involved."[25] Effective disaster preparedness must recognize that disaster health care occurs within a disaster setting, where social structures have been damaged or are of lesser standards than accustomed, because disaster by definition is a "serious disruption of the functioning of a community or society, causing widespread human, material, economic or environmental losses which exceed the ability of the affected community or society to cope using only its own resources."[26]

The importance of and dependence on infrastructural systems for societal functioning and disaster recovery has been recognized by national and international preparedness and response agencies (**Table 2**). Nurses in this study did not anticipate for their health care response to be impacted by the lessened capabilities of these health-care-enabling systems during a disaster event. Nurses from other countries

---

Box 5
Nurses' statements regarding disaster preparedness and knowledge

RN1: And one of the lessons learned, ... that I am vividly aware of, is that ... the immediate disaster response time in those shelters is not the time to initiate a detox program.

RN2: A lot of times I see emergency management, they have to have their drills, that's how they get their money, and so they want 'em done by 4:30.

RN2: "I can do like 10 people with their blood pressure medicine or one person with human immunodeficiency virus," and he was seeing the light that there was gonna be an ethical dilemma for him... because ... he was gonna have to choose who got their medicines.

RN3: Most of the nurses ... have this mistaken belief that they are coming to fix trauma and it's gonna be exciting and it's gonna be lights and sirens. ... They have that mistaken belief because ...the systems perpetuate that belief that that's what nursing is in disaster. ... Nurses coming into disaster are led to believe by the systems that disaster work is trauma based. Nurses leave disaster nursing once they figure it out that it is public health work, not acute and trauma based. ... Ninety percent public health nurses, 10% acute needed. You flip the current model in disaster. And, frankly, we need to flip the current model in nursing education the way we're going in our health care system. But I think if the – if we can get the education flipped for the health care system training, then we will be better in disaster. We will....This is what you need in disaster, not the high-tech stuff.

RN4: We prepared ... how to use the fire extinguisher, put the fire out, but we didn't prepare on how to prevent the fire in the first place.

RN5: It just was something that none of us had ever gone through before and we learned.

RN6: I'm a nurse but it was actually a very small piece of what's going on in the grand spectrum of things, and it was learning the cultures and ... what I have to work with and what I don't have to work with are even bigger.

RN7: Everyone knows to go to the command center so that you have a starting point for communication. You just don't know that the command center's not gonna have power and it's in a structure...with gases that are leaking and... it's not a structure that they want to let people enter into.

RN8: The nurses themselves ... had to fall back and think more on their medical/surgical training as a nurse... Uh, and I think it's wonderful that we do have the specialties; however, um, I think sometimes because you get so far away from your basic medical/surgical training that you don't think along those lines. ...They don't tend to think along the lines of a medical nurse....

RN9: I didn't know what to expect.

RN10: The level of inexperience [of nurses] was a continual challenge.

RN11: We couldn't do a lot of our interventions 'cause we didn't have stuff.

---

have also experienced similar unexpected physical, structural, climatologic, cultural, and clinical disaster conditions.[27–30]

Fundamentals of Health Care

Although some nurses suggest "the skills required in disaster are the same as those required on a regular shift,"[31] nurses in this study primarily used first aid, basic assessment, nursing fundamentals, and population health skills while caring for survivors. These findings concur with the disaster experiences described by nurses worldwide.[1,27,32–34]

Vulnerable Populations

Despite an average of 25 years of nursing experience, nurses in this study seemed surprised by the diversity of people they encountered during their disaster responses,

Table 2 Organization-specific critical societal sectors	
US National Response Framework (Department of Homeland Security, 2013).	**United Nations Cluster Approach (Inter-Agency Standing Committee, 2012).**
Transportation	Health
Communication	Emergency shelter
Public works and engineering	Water, sanitation, and hygiene
Firefighting	Logistics
Emergency management	Camp coordination and management
Mass care	Protection
Emergency assistance	Nutrition
Housing and human services	Food security
Search and rescue	Emergency telecommunications
Oil and hazardous materials response	Education
Agriculture and natural resources	Early recovery
Energy	
Public safety and security	
External affairs	

especially those seeking assistance in disaster clinics and shelters. The unexpected survivor groups that "stood out" and were explicitly named by the nurses in this study are otherwise known as "vulnerable populations," or groups who have been habitually neglected and underserved by society and government.[35] Already carrying a larger burden of ill health in US society,[36] vulnerable populations are more susceptible to harm, and thus most in need following disaster.[37]

The needs of vulnerable populations are not being sufficiently considered during disaster planning and response.[38] Municipalities have been found guilty of "benign neglect" and in violation of US civil rights legislation for not recognizing and properly planning for population vulnerabilities during disaster.[39] A comprehensive emergency preparedness framework was recently created because efforts by hospital and emergency planners to include "the needs of vulnerable populations...have lagged."[40] Implicit racial bias has been demonstrated in nursing faculty[41] and primary care providers.[42] An Emergency Nurses Association board member just called for compassion by emergency nurses toward the homeless and "to take interest in this forgotten population."[43] To halt further neglect of at-risk populations during disaster, nurses must be prepared to encounter and address the specialized health care needs of these neglected groups.

Environmental Influence on Health Outcomes

A person's health, functioning, and quality-of-life outcomes and risks are affected by where one is born, lives, and works.[44] It follows that the living and working environment of nurses may affect their health, functioning, and quality of life outcomes.

Nurses in this study attributed their emotional distress to their exposure to the human and physical devastation of the disaster environment. In the emergency department, stress has been associated with emergency nurses' constant exposure to acute and traumatic patients[45] and the "challenges" of ... "unreliable technology" and "insufficient hospital resources" for "high patient volumes."[46]

Anticipating unfavorable hospital working conditions, nurses worldwide report a lack of intention to report to work during disaster.[47–50] In survivors, stress has been associated with living in their damaged environment.[51] It must be considered that the disrupted conditions of the disaster environmental may also be contributing to distress in nurses following their disaster experiences.

Preparedness

All nurses are expected to be properly prepared for a disaster response.[52] However, the "sporadic nature of disaster nursing education has resulted in a workforce with limited capability to respond in the event of a disaster, develop policy, educate or accept leadership roles. ... The risk is further increased by hesitancy to respond as a result of a lack of knowledge."[52]

Nurses worldwide share a belief that "nothing had prepared" them for the conditions they encountered during their disaster response.[1,29,53,54] Hospital MCI training was "totally different" than US nurses' actual experience volunteering postdisaster at a community shelter.[55] Disaster-experienced nurses support the need for better disaster education.[29,53] Nurses ill-prepared for environmental conditions of disaster may become victims instead, adding to the scope of the disaster.[56]

IMPLICATIONS

Stress may be reduced through preparedness for the expected condition,[57] thus preparation for the likely environmental conditions surrounding a disaster health care response may reduce stress in nurses. The inherent loss of resources during disaster and the subsequent effects on health care capabilities are not currently part of disaster nursing education, training, or research.

Implications for Nursing Education

Preparedness for disaster health care should become an extension of regular health care, and nursing education should emphasize population and public health skills over acute and trauma-centered hospital care in every day care and during disaster. A population approach would also address the embedded physical, economic, and social conditions that differentially affect vulnerable populations, and prepare nurses to serve those populations most at risk following a disaster. Additionally, first aid certification should be required of all nurses.

Implications for Clinical Practice

Nursing preparedness protocols, education, and training should anticipate damage and interruptions to health care's supporting infrastructure. Nurses should expect to provide care with limited technology and medical supplies, and focus instead on basics of physiology and population health.

Individually, nurses must assess their own readiness for deployment, and their comfort with rudimentary living situations, along with their physical conditioning for the arduous and physically demanding workload and conditions. Several organizations provide training and field orientation to prepare health care workers for the non–health care contexts of disaster response.[58–60] These broader disaster environment topics could be readily incorporated into current disaster preparedness plans and training.

Implications for Future Research

Further qualitative studies are needed to identify the full set of contextual variables of the disaster environment that impact nurses' ability to provide nursing care. The relationship between these environmental aspects with adverse psychosocial effects in disaster nurses should also be investigated. Identifying the environmental components nurses were and were not prepared for is also needed. There is a suggestion in the literature that nurses already familiar with low-resource settings may be better prepared for the disaster settings,[5,61] and this should be pursued. Disaster nursing competencies should be assessed for comprehensiveness, and include competencies for living and working in the altered conditions of the disaster environment.

SUMMARY

Nurses described the difficult health care setting and broader environmental challenges they experienced during their disaster experiences. These "not normal" disaster conditions contrasted greatly with these nurses' normal nursing training, expectations, behavior, and actions. US nursing education, preparedness drills, and disaster competencies rarely anticipate the loss of structural systems that support the health care system following a disaster event.

Preparing nurses for the likely reductions in health care supplies and equipment along with the reduced capabilities of society's supportive infrastructure during disaster may lessen the detrimental effects of disaster deployments on nurses, improve survivor care following disaster, and increase the retention of disaster-experienced nurses in the ranks of health professions following a disaster deployment.

Limitations

This study was limited to US nurses, and suffers from a lack of diversity in the study population. Elapsed time since their experience may have moderated participants' disaster recollections. Nurses with relevant disaster experience may have been excluded from this study because of military status or withdrawal from the nursing profession.

REFERENCES

1. Jordan-Welch ML. "Nursing in hell": the experience of providing care during and after Hurricane Katrina: nursing. 2007.
2. Klein KR, Nagel NE. Mass medical evacuation: Hurricane Katrina and nursing experiences at the New Orleans airport. Disaster Manag Response 2007;5(2): 56–61.
3. Rivers FM. Into the unknown: military nurses' experiences in disasters response [dissertation]. Knoxville (TN): University of Tennessee; 2009.
4. Sloand E, Ho G, Klimmek R, et al. Nursing children after a disaster: a qualitative study of nurse volunteers and children after the Haiti earthquake. J Spec Pediatr Nurs 2012;17(3):242–53.
5. Fink S. Five days at memorial. New York: Crown Publishers; 2013.
6. Tomer J. Into the ruins: nurses in Haiti. Minor Nurse News. 2010. Available at: http://www.minoritynurse.com/article/ruins-nurses-haiti. Accessed June 29, 2013.
7. Leiby SL. Caring for the caregivers and patients left behind: experiences of a volunteer nurse during Hurricane Katrina. Crit Care Nurs Clin North Am 2008; 20(1):83–90.
8. Bless M. Thoughts on serving: two weeks as a post-hurricane volunteer. 2005. Available at: http://medscapenursing.blogs.com/medscape_nursing/hurricane_katrina_nurses_and_nps_help/. Accessed August 4, 2013.
9. Marshall MC. San Antonio Mental Health Disaster Consortium: Hurricanes Katrina and Rita, a personal perspective. Perspect Psychiatr Care 2007;43(1):15–21.

10. VanDevanter N, Kovner CT, Raveis VH, et al. Challenges of nurses' deployment to other New York City hospitals in the aftermath of Hurricane Sandy. J Urban Health 2014;91(4):603–14.
11. Park WH. Nurses' posttraumatic stress, level of exposure, and coping five years after Hurricane Katrina [dissertation]. Atlanta (GA): Georgia State University; 2011.
12. Zhen Y, Huang ZQ, Jin J, et al. Post-traumatic stress disorder of red cross nurses in the aftermath of the 2008 Wenchuan China Earthquake. Arch Psychiatr Nurs 2012;26(1):63–70.
13. Boswell S. I saved the iguana: a mixed methods study examining responder mental health after major disasters and humanitarian relief events [dissertation]. Knoxville (TN): University of Tennessee; 2014.
14. Laube J. Psychological reactions of nurses in disaster. Nurs Res 1973;22(4): 343–7.
15. Palm KM, Polusny MA, Follette VM. Vicarious traumatization: potential hazards and interventions for disaster and trauma workers. Prehosp Disaster Med 2004; 19(1):73–8.
16. Urrabazo CK. Anxiety, coping, and post-traumatic stress disorder in nurses who cared for victims of Hurricane Katrina [dissertation]. Denton (TX): Texas Woman's University; 2012.
17. Morse JM. Introducing the first global congress for qualitative health research: what are we? What will we do? -And why? Qual Health Res 2012;22(2):147–56.
18. Brink PJ, Wood MJ. Advanced design in nursing research. 2nd edition. Thousand Oaks (CA): Sage Publications; 1998.
19. Merleau-Ponty M. The primacy of perception. Evanston (IL): Northwestern University Press; 1964.
20. Thomas SP, Pollio HR. Listening to patients: a phenomenological approach to nursing research and practice. New York: Springer Publishing; 2002.
21. Creswell JW. Research design: qualitative, quantitative, and mixed methods approaches. Los Angeles (CA): Sage Publications; 2009.
22. Creswell JW. Qualitative inquiry and research design: choosing among five approaches. Washington, DC: Sage Publications, Inc; 2013.
23. Guest G, Bunce A, Johnson L. How many interviews are enough?: an experiment with data saturation and variability. Field Meth 2006;18:59–82.
24. Lincoln YS, Guba EG. Naturalistic inquiry. Beverly Hills (CA): Sage Publications; 1985.
25. al-Madhari AF, Keller AZ. Review of disaster definitions. Prehosp Disaster Med 1997;12(1):17–20.
26. Inter-Agency Standing Committee. 2009 UNISDR terminology on disaster risk reduction. 2009. Available at: http://www.unisdr.org/files/7817_UNISDRTermino logyEnglish.pdf. Accessed March 1, 2015.
27. Richardson S, Ardagh M, Grainger P, et al. A moment in time: emergency nurses and the Canterbury earthquakes. Int Nurs Rev 2013;60(2):188–95.
28. Nasrabadi AN, Naji H, Mirzabeigi G, et al. Earthquake relief: Iranian nurses' responses in Bam, 2003, and lessons learned. Int Nurs Rev 2007;54(1):13–8.
29. Wenji Z, Turale S, Stone TE, et al. Chinese nurses' relief experiences following two earthquakes: implications for disaster education and policy development. Nurse Educ Pract 2014;15:75–81.
30. Kayama M, Akiyama T, Ohashi A, et al. Experiences of municipal public health nurses following Japan's earthquake, tsunami, and nuclear disaster. Public Health Nurs 2014;31(6):517–25.

31. Gebbie KM, Hutton A, Plummer V. Update on competencies and education. Annu Rev Nurs Res 2012;30:169–92.
32. Ruskie SE. Nurses' perceptions of environment as a factor in their capacity to provide effective disaster care: pilot study. Paper presented at the 19th World Congress on Disaster and Emergency Medicine. Capetown, South Africa, April 22, 2015.
33. Ruskie SE. "You came to not normal land": Nurses' experience of the environment of disaster [dissertation]. Knoxville (TN): University of Tennessee; 2015.
34. Redwood-Campbell LJ, Riddez L. Post-tsunami medical care: health problems encountered in the International Committee of the Red Cross hospital in Banda Aceh, Indonesia. Prehosp Disaster Med 2006;21(Suppl 1):S1–7.
35. Warren RC, Walker B Jr, Maclin SD Jr, et al. Respecting and protecting the beloved community, especially susceptible and vulnerable populations. J Health Care Poor Underserved 2011;22(Suppl 3):3–13.
36. Institute of Medicine. Unequal treatment: confronting racial and ethnic disparities in health care. Washington, DC: National Academies Press; 2002.
37. Powers R, Daly E, editors. International disaster nursing. New York: Cambridge University Press; 2010.
38. Flanagan BE, Gregory EW, Hallisey EJ, et al. A social vulnerability index for disaster management. J Homel Secur Emerg Manag 2011;8(1):1–22.
39. Santora M, Weiser B. Court says New York neglected disabled in emergencies. New York Times 2013.
40. Kreisberg D, Thomas DSK, Valley M, et al. Vulnerable populations in hospital and health care emergency preparedness planning: a comprehensive framework for inclusion. Prehosp Disaster Med 2016;31(2):211–9.
41. Fitzsimmons KA. The existence of implicit racial bias in nursing faculty [dissertation]. Greeley (CO): University of Northern Colorado; 2009.
42. Blair IV, Havranek EP, Price DW, et al. Assessment of biases against Latinos and African Americans among primary care providers and community members. Am J Public Health 2013;103(1):92–8.
43. Solheim J. A call for compassion toward the homeless. ENA Connection 2016; 40(3):8.
44. U.S. Department of Health and Human Services. Healthy People 2020. 2012. Available at: http://www.healthypeople.gov/2020/default.aspx.
45. Duffy E, Avalos G, Dowling M. Secondary traumatic stress among emergency nurses: a cross-sectional study. Int Emerg Nurs 2015;23(2):53–8.
46. Wolf LA, Perhats C, Delao AM, et al. "It's a burden you carry": describing moral distress in emergency nursing. J Emerg Nurs 2016;42(1):37–46.
47. Arbon P, Cusack L, Ranse J, et al. Exploring staff willingness to attend work during a disaster: a study of nurses employed in four Australian emergency departments. Australas Emerg Nurs J 2013;16(3):103–9.
48. Connor SB. Factors associated with the intention of health care personnel to respond to a disaster. Prehosp Disaster Med 2014;29(6):555–60.
49. Melnikov S, Itzhaki M, Kagan I. Israeli nurses' intention to report for work in an emergency or disaster. J Nurs Scholarsh 2014;46(2):134–42.
50. O'Boyle C, Robertson C, Secor-Turner M. Nurses' beliefs about public health emergencies: fear of abandonment. Am J Infect Control 2006;34(6):351–7.
51. Warsini S, Buettner P, Mills J, et al. The psychosocial impact of the environmental damage caused by the Mt. Merapi eruption on survivors in Indonesia. Ecohealth 2014;11(4):491–501.
52. World Health Organization and International Council of Nurses. ICN framework of disaster nurse competencies. Geneva (Switzerland): WHO; 2009.

53. Yang YN, Xiao LD, Cheng HY, et al. Chinese nurses' experience in the Wenchuan earthquake relief. Int Nurs Rev 2010;57(2):217–23.

54. Sloand E, Ho G, Kub J. Experiences of nurse volunteers in Haiti after the 2010 earthquake. Res Theory Nurs Pract 2013;27(3):193–213.

55. Shipman SJ, Stanton MP, Tomlinson S, et al. Qualitative analysis of the lived experience of first-time nurse responders in disaster. J Contin Educ Nurs 2016;47(2): 61–71.

56. Van Hoving DJ, Wallis LA, Docrat F, et al. Haiti disaster tourism: a medical shame. Prehosp Disaster Med 2010;25(3):201–2.

57. Glass DC, Singer JE. Urban stress: Experiments on noise and social stressors. New York: Academic Press; 1972.

58. Global Emergency Group. Humanitarian Field Training. 2016. Available at: http://globalemergencygroup.com/files/GEG%20Humanitarian%20Field%20Training%20May%2020-24%202013%284%29.pdf.

59. RedR UK. Find a training course. 2016. Available at: http://www.redr.org.uk/en/Training-and-more/find-a-training-course.cfm.

60. Medair. Field selection and orientation. 2016. Available at: http://relief.medair.org/en/jobs/field-selection-and-orientation/.

61. Kawano R. Answering Katrina's call. Minor Nurse News. 2006. Available at: http://minoritynurse.com/answering-katrinas-call/. Accessed June 29, 2013.

Complicated Realities
Mental Health and Moral Incongruence
in Disaster/Humanitarian Response

Suzanne M. Boswell, PhD, MSN, RN, CCRA*

KEYWORDS

- Moral incongruence • Psychological stress • Ethics • Humanitarian • Disaster

KEY POINTS

- Moral complexity, an inherent characteristic within disaster/humanitarian settings, has an impact on responder mental health.
- An individual serving as a disaster ethicist has the potential to make a valuable contribution to moral decision-making and potentially decrease responders' psychological burden.
- Providing care within differing cultural settings creates additional uncertainty when weighing right or wrong responses to morally complex questions.

INTRODUCTION

The setting is austere, and victims arrive in greater numbers as search and rescue efforts intensify. The number of patients is overwhelming. Exhausted due to inability to sleep, extended 14-hour to 16-hour workdays, and hot temperatures, decisions allocating and rationing limited resources are made reflexively. Time and energy to rationalize and reflect on thought processes is scarce. In the quiet moments, my decisions return to haunt me, and I struggle with my decisions in angst.

The scenario is derived from the experiences of one who worked diligently to restore a modicum of stability to Haitian residents after the January 12, 2010, earthquake.[1] Although this scenario is reflective of one responder's dilemma, stories of moral distress among disaster/humanitarian responders are common.

Morality is inherently intertwined into the organization of social practices.[2] Exploration of press releases, research, blog entries, and other documentation of disaster/humanitarian events reveal that morality and ethics are also woven into the social contract between responders and survivors. In fact, the International Red Cross Code of

Disclosure Statement: The author listed above has no commercial or professional affiliation with an institution that has a financial interest on the topic disclosed herein.
University of Tennessee College of Nursing, 1200 Volunteer Boulevard, Knoxville, TN 37996, USA
* 11 Thunder Bay Drive, Johnson City, TN 37615.
E-mail address: Suz2012@comcast.net

Conduct for the International Red Cross and Red Crescent Movement and nongovernmental organizations (NGOs) in disaster relief (**Box 1**) asserts that the motivation of disaster response is to relieve human suffering in a manner that is neither partisan nor politically or religiously motivated. Likewise, responders are to strive to assuage human suffering in recognition that life is to be valued without consideration to geographic boundaries.[3]

Due to the nature of disaster/humanitarian work, the extent to which disaster/humanitarian responders can and do apply basic ethical principles (**Box 2**)[4–6] to moral decision-making processes is not known.[7,8] In the course of disaster/humanitarian response, providers are exposed to chaotic environments riddled with morally complex situations. Humanitarian work has been described as a morally complex activity characterized by family and friends who are geographically distant, extended work hours, ethically charged dilemmas, rapid change, and volatility mixed with intervals of tedium and routine. Consequently, responders immersed in the milieu may perform activities that result in unintended harm.[9]

In disaster settings, psychological trauma may be exacerbated by visual cues while working among the dead or grossly injured, risk of personal injury, extended work hours, individual and group suffering, moral distress as a result of alterations to normal practice in the provision of care, and extended chaos.[9–11] Moreover, forces within the responder's organization or response team have the power to push values that normally affect personal behavior into the background.[12] For these reasons, disaster/humanitarian responders, who are immersed in efforts to mitigate poverty, suffering, and death, are often confronted with morally complex situations.

Moral incongruence may occur as responders, accustomed to providing individualized care, reorient their thinking to provide population-based care in the face of insufficient supplies, inadequate infrastructure, and lack of trained personnel.[6,8] Resource allocation in austere settings is a factor in moral compromise among

---

Box 1
Code of conduct for the International Red Cross and Red Crescent Movement and nongovernmental organizations in disaster relief

1. The humanitarian imperative comes first.

2. Aid is given regardless of race, creed, or nationality of the recipients and without adverse distinction of any kind. Aid priorities are calculated on the basis of need alone.

3. Aid will not be used to further a particular political or religious standpoint.

4. We shall endeavor not to act as instruments of governmental foreign policy.

5. We shall respect culture and custom.

6. We shall attempt to build disaster response on local capabilities.

7. Ways shall be found to involve program beneficiaries in the management of relief aid.

8. Relief aid must strive to reduce future vulnerabilities to disaster as well as meeting basic needs.

9. We hold ourselves accountable to both those we seek to assist and those from whom we accept resources.

10. In our information, publicity, and advertising activities, we shall recognize disaster victims as dignified human beings, not hopeless objects.

From the International Federation of Red Cross and Red Crescent Societies, 25 May, 2016; with permission.

Box 2
Basic ethical principles

- Beneficence
  - Ethical treatment of individuals through respect for their decisions, protection from harm, and efforts to secure safety and well-being.
- Nonmaleficence
  - Provision of care in a manner that does not result in harm or hurt.
- Justice
  - Ensures that people receive benefits to which they are entitled rather than having them denied without good reason, thus imposing unreasonable burden.
- Respect for persons
  - Recognizes that people must be recognized as autonomous agents. Individuals who cannot act autonomously are entitled to protection.
- Fidelity
  - Provision of care that incorporates actions of loyalty, fairness, truthfulness, advocacy, and commitment.
- Paternalism
  - Opposes the principle of autonomy in that providers assume the role of decision-maker and treat individuals based on personal belief about what is best for the recipient of care.

---

disaster/humanitarian responders. Application of the ethical principle of distributive justice is hampered by lack of empirical evidence to guide providers who must rely on values-based decision-making in an effort to ensure equity among the surviving.[13–15] Crisis Standards of Care (CSC)[16] includes a recommendation that health care workers maintain ethical and professional standards in CSC. Among these principles are duty to steward resources, fairness, and duty to care.

In many cases, strategic stockpiles and sharing resources among communities are inadequate to meet response needs. Awareness of the ethical implications of lack of essential supplies to respond is present at individual, organizational, and federal levels.[15] In determining who will receive and benefit from available resources, providers must consider fairness and nondiscriminatory practice, the legality of the decision, and parameters of current policy.[13] The mental health burden of responder guilt due to perceptions of insufficient response as a result of scarcity of resources is pervasive.[7,17] Despite this, responders must provide the best care possible with minimal resources.

Additionally, accounts of the responder experience reveal opportunities for individuals to perform tasks outside their current scope of practice. Guides to practice, such as training, licensing boards, and professional ethical behavior in traditional settings, may be supplanted in the humanitarian field, thus altering the way that responders cope with ethical dilemmas.[18] Although decision-making processes meld practical wisdom, and detail to determine a course of action,[19] moral conflict may arise as responders strive to determine the acceptability of performing tasks outside the normal scope of practice.

Four moral values appear consistently within the ranks of humanitarian workers: preservation of human life; human rights defined by the spectrum of values across economic, political, social, and civil domains; justice demonstrated by fair and equal relationships between individuals and groups within a society; and staff safety. Moral dilemmas leading to disputes over human life versus human freedom may occur when these principles are not prioritized consistently among organizations and individual responders.[20]

Mental health of disaster/humanitarian responders is instrumental in well-being and retention of seasoned responders best equipped to provide care to communities in times of urgent need. Inexperienced responders may be unprepared for resource scarcity and conflicts between organizational policy and local laws. As with experienced responders, they may experience moral distress from incongruence in the application of ethical principles. Ultimately, a reduction in responder human resources compromises success in response efforts.

A number of concepts are used in an effort to place a label on the psychological burden of moral compromise. Among them are moral distress, which is defined as uncomfortable psychological disequilibrium that occurs as a result of unethical performance due to obstacles such as time, supervisory conflict, legal parameters, organizational policy, and hierarchical relationships.[21] Moral injury, defined as psychological stress occurring as a result of a violation to deeply held moral and ethical beliefs and expectations by self or others, was assessed by Nash and colleagues[22] in an effort to develop an instrument to assist with identifying causes of moral distress in veterans. Indeed, a debate about the most appropriate conceptual term for this stress-inducing phenomenon is ongoing.[23] Likewise, the complex relationship between ethics and psychological health is multifaceted because determinations about right versus wrong, and moral versus immoral decisions and activities are as diverse as the values held by the individuals performing responder tasks. Consequently, this article is not intended to render an opinion about ideal terminology, but to inform the reader about the impact of ethical dilemmas on the mental health of disaster/humanitarian responders. Within this article, moral incongruence is used as an overarching term to address both internal and external constraints on moral decision-making and ethical behavior.

Research examining the effects of the response experience on mental health is growing, but specific influences are not well explored. The purpose of this article was to disseminate research findings that highlight the impact of moral incongruence on responder mental health within the disaster/humanitarian setting by focusing on the theme "Everything was gray." The information is extracted from a larger, mixed methods study examining numerous variables considered within relevant literature to be influential in the occurrence of psychological distress among disaster/humanitarian responders.[24] Due to space limitations, complete findings of the study are not included herewith.

METHODS
Ethics Approval

Assurance that this research was performed according to ethical guidelines was essential for the protection of disaster/humanitarian responders who volunteered their time and sharing of their story so freely to facilitate greater understanding of the response experience. This research was approved by an institutional review board before obtaining informed consent and initiation of study procedures.

Study Sample

The sample for phenomenological exploration of the experience of disaster response was composed of 10 volunteers who agreed to participate following completion of an online survey. The sample consisted of 1 mental health worker, 2 physicians, 2 firemen/emergency medical technicians (EMTs), 1 EMT, 2 paramedics, and 2 nurses. Experiences of the participants included both man-made and natural disasters, including the 2013 Boston Marathon bombings, Typhoon Haiyan, the 2010 Haitian Earthquake, Hurricane Katrina, settings of massive fires that displaced hundreds of victims, and chemical spills requiring survivor evacuation. **Table 1** provides an introduction to the participants. Profession has been combined with the most memorable response event so as to provide an identifier.

Data Analysis

All interviews were recorded and transcribed by the researcher. Thereafter, they were de-identified for data analysis. Analysis of the interviews was performed according to the method detailed by Thomas and Pollio.[25] All interviews were read line by line so as to obtain an overview of each participant's story. Thereafter, each story was read again to identify recurring words, phrases, or ideas. These items were determined to be meaningful in the disaster/humanitarian response experience, and they serve as the base on which themes were established. Themes derived from the meaning units are descriptive and stated in the words of the participants. It is from these themes that the thematic structure, a visually descriptive representation of the study findings, emerged.

FINDINGS

Qualitative findings include the themes of "I lost my footing," "I saw everything was gray," "I was totally vulnerable," "That's why I do it," and "I get to go home." The first theme represents chaos, the contextual ground on which the responder experience occurs. The second lends itself to a description of the experience of altered expectations that occurs during the response. A story of feelings of vulnerability unfolds with the fourth theme, and an understanding of the reasons responders are willing to engage themselves for others is told in "That's why I do it." The theme "I saw everything was gray" is the focus of this article, and it is broken down in to smaller, subthemes so as to extricate the moral components that impacted the mental health of participants.

"I Saw Everything Was Gray"

The color gray is a somber hue that represents the ambiguity that is characteristic of disaster/humanitarian response activities. In the response setting, traditional

Table 1 Study sample		
Participant	**Gender**	**Country of Origin**
MD: Hurricane Katrina	Male	USA
MD: Typhoon Haiyan	Female	Philippines
Mental Health Worker: Haiti Earthquake	Female	USA
RN: Boston Marathon Bombing	Female	USA
RN: Cambodian Refugee Crisis	Female	USA
Paramedic: Hurricane Katrina	Male	USA
Paramedic: Chemical Explosion	Male	Canada
EMT: Hurricane Katrina	Male	USA
Fireman/EMT: Hurricane Sandy	Female	USA
Fireman/EMT: California Wildfire	Male	USA

Abbreviations: EMT, emergency medical technician; MD, medical doctor; RN, registered nurse.

standards of care must be altered due to austere settings. Plans formulated before arrival often require modification to meet survivors' needs. Disaster/humanitarian events are replete with uncertainty, right or wrong answers to health care dilemmas in these settings may be evasive.

I was so earnest, and I thought I had it all figured out. And then I got there, and everything was gray. All of my instructions had to go out the window.
—Registered nurse (RN): Cambodian Refugee Crisis

Sometimes I thought, Did I make the right choice? Could that have been done better? Could it have been done faster?
—Fireman/EMT: California Wildfire

"Did I Ever Think I Was Meant to Save the Life of an Iguana?"

Disaster/humanitarian events are replete with uncertainty, and there may be no right or wrong answers to ethical dilemmas in these settings. Uncertainty is difficult to cope with when decisions may result in life or death. Respect for life is integral to the responder role, and the ultimate goal is to ensure well-being of the living. Responders shared memories of lives encountered. Ultimately, preservation, like loss, can be neither guaranteed or understood.

… did I ever think I was meant to save the life of an iguana by breaking out a hot pack and putting it on him because there was no heat lamp? No, but I did one time.
—RN: Boston Marathon Bombing

Now, one of the houses that we were protecting, we were standing on a ridgeline in between a valley and the house, and I felt something nudge up against the inside of one of my boots, and it was a rabbit. And this rabbit was basically huddled up against me, and it looked up at me, and then I looked back down, and it took off down the hill and ran into the fire. Now, I thought it was extremely odd that this would happen. It's something that even to this day, on the very rare occasion that I do think about it, I mean, you know, really? What the hell? You know, you—you come running up, you lay against my boot, and then you run down the hill into the fire lines.
—Fireman/EMT: California Wildfire

"Complicated Realities"

Unlike traditional health care settings, efforts to ensure the safety and well-being of survivors may compete with a goal for personal safety. In moments of potential personal danger and risk, turning away from those you endeavor to protect and serve may produce emotions and actions that run counter to self-preservation or goals of deployment.

….and the alarm sounded and they started rounding up all of the aid workers and responders. And they said, "We have to leave and go to a rendezvous point away from the border as quickly as possible. We're expecting bombing of the camp." And there was a nurse there from Australia, and she wrapped herself around one of the poles in the middle of the makeshift hospital and refused to leave. And they kept trying and trying to bring her away and she said, "No, I'm not leaving these people. What's gonna happen to them?" And that's one of the complicated realities, that in a life-threatening situation we had the option to run away.
—RN: Cambodian Refugee Crisis

Well, you know, nobody likes to get shot at. I guess if you think back on that, part of you is pissed off about, you know, Seriously, dude? We're here trying to help you out and you're shooting at us? Thanks for that! It makes you angry a bit. It's frustrating sometimes, to see the way people behave sometimes. You know, there's the folks who try to help themselves and, and help their neighbors and do what you think is the right thing; and there's others who are busy looting whatever they can get ahold of and taking advantage of the situation. And, you know, that's, that's irritating and frustrating and makes you angry.

—*Medical doctor (MD): Hurricane Katrina*

"It Was the Right Thing to Do"

Decisions must be made within the dichotomy of right and wrong, and it is likely that no two responders will make the same decision as a result of differing cultural influences, values, experience levels, codes of conduct, and numerous contextual factors. The *right* action may be illusive, and the impact on responders' mental health has the potential to produce long-term remorse.

You know, sort of according to our codes of conduct, I knew that it [saving a woman's life] was the right thing to do, as a professional, and I always wondered was it the right thing to do for her. And there's no way you can ever know that. That was one of those ambiguous events in life that you just have to live with. You look around, and you see the circumstances and you know, she just made that determination about her life. And here I come with completely different cultural context and disrupt that. You know, women were not always treated well. You know, who knows what grief she was living with, what she had been through and witnessed....But there we were together.

—*RN: Cambodian Refugee Crisis*

"You Use What You Got Available"

In traditional settings, supplies to provide care are most always available or can be ordered via telephone or electronic medical record system. In austere settings, supplies are not always readily available, and responders are often in need of items to restore health or provide comfort. Inability to meet basic needs of survivors results in a burdensome realization that the medical system in place was ineffective despite the energy expended.

A lot of things in EMS are just kind of McGyvering it; I mean, if it doesn't work, you've gotta find something that works.

—*Fireman/EMT: Hurricane Sandy*

Of course, primarily you pity them and then you wish you could have brought some more, like, a simple tetanus vaccine. So after a week, the [medical] system didn't work. We started getting patients who were already having tetanus. Like this one man, he was a patient; he was already having spasms, one of the signs of tetanus, and it could have been prevented by just being able to give him the necessary medicine. When we went to that next town, we were also looking for tetanus vaccines. But we went to all the pharmacies, but we didn't find any more.

—*MD: Typhoon Haiyan*

There was a major suicide attempt, and a lady slit both her arms and both wrists with a barber's razor in a tent, on an air mattress in a tent and took 6 bottles of pills. We were using 39-gallon trash can bag liners to put over her arms and legs and to

apply pressure and stop the bleeding. You use what you got available, and you use it. The supplies were somewhere, but they weren't in the tents… And, you know, just in the real world you gotta' just do what you do in the real world.
— RN: Boston Marathon Bombing

"I Hate Feeling Helpless"

Acknowledging responders' reverence for the sanctity of life, the difficulty in coping with feelings of helplessness, helplessness to preserve life and restore well-being, cannot be disregarded. As one responder informed me, helplessness prompts worthlessness, and the emotion directly contradicts the response effort to do more, not just do enough to assist survivors.

I'm sorry I can't get to you. I can't help you because your house is surrounded in 15 foot of saltwater. I'm sorry I can't get to you because your house was leveled, and I can't get to you. You had pre-warning to get out. But you chose to stay, and now you want me to come in the middle of the storm and get you. Yeah, that's, that's difficult to, for anybody's problem. You know, how would anybody cope with that? You know, how do they expect, you try to get there but you can't do it, you just can't get there. Helplessness. Number one, first and foremost. And that's a feeling I hate. I hate feeling helpless. That, that is, that's the easiest way to put it, I feel helpless. And when you feel helpless you feel almost worthless because you know that you're trying to get there and there's nothing you can do to get there.
— EMT: Hurricane Katrina

Anger, guilt. Occasionally, hell, not a feeling of worthlessness but feeling like you could have done more, regardless of what anybody tells you.
— Fire/EMT: California Wildfires

"We Have This Inherent Need to Fix Things… Be Sure It's Permanent"

In their effort to do more, to care more than enough, lies responders' desire to be assured that their labor will have a long-term, positive impact on survivors and their communities. Uncertainty of the future brings knowledge that there is no guarantee of stability for survivors. Participants spoke emotionally about abandoning expectations that survivors and communities would be restored to normalcy after the response. In reality, the result of a responder's labor may be only temporary due to circumstances over which they cannot exert control. This is in conflict with an internal desire to facilitate long-term recovery, and the unmet goal may precipitate feelings of remorse.

We have this inherent need to fix things, rescue people, and be sure it sticks, be sure it's permanent. And it was real hard to let go of that man because I knew he was going back out on the streets at his preference. And all that assistance would probably fall by the wayside. That was a difficult thing to let go of.
— RN: North Dakota Floods

One of the hardest things at the beginning was that a few people came in that had a bad situation, a bad life before the disaster, and then a disaster hit, and they're gonna have a bad life after. They didn't have any money before the storm, and they're not gonna have any money after the storm, and now they don't have a house either. So we're there to fix and help with their immediate disaster-related needs, but we can't fix their whole life. We're there to put a Band-Aid on what the storm did to that part of their life, and that's what we can do. So to make decisions like that ... you have to say "no" on some things. You would love to be able to give 'em everything they need, but you can't.

—RN: Hurricane Katrina

"There's No One to Call"

Responders informed me that they are often faced with challenging decisions for which they have no one to consult to obtain a response. Similarly, they may be witness to the unjust and mustering inner strength, serve to provide a voice for those who succumb to injustice in the midst of recovery. In either case, the emotional toll takes physical and mental energy to mitigate morally incongruent events.

Oh, God, like when you're in a situation where you've got to make difficult decisions, or you've made a difficult decision and then you have to live with it, to have somebody kind of walk through that with you would be helpful. When you have a moral conflict, you, there's no one, no one to pick up and call for somebody to help you out there...even in Katrina, you have to decide who's gonna get medical care and who isn't.

—RN: Cambodian Refugee Crisis

You know, there were all these chemical plants along the river down there. I think that's the gulf. And so they came in and they got up on the stage and they said, you know, "Anybody that wants work," you know, "come with us and we'll pay you 10 dollars an hour." And people were practically fainting. That was like a fortune. They had never made 10 dollars an hour before. Many volunteers who went off, mostly young people, you know, sitting in the shelter is boring, there's nothing to do. But then, they started showing up with terrible, like rashes and coughs and some GI upsets. So after talking to them, it became very clear that they were being exposed to chemicals without any training, without the proper protective equipment. Plus, they weren't getting paid the money that they were owed. First of all, it just infuriated me that anybody would come in and exploit these people who had already been through Katrina....There were 2 police officers who came from the local police force. I said, "You know, people are going off, doing this work, and they're coming back and they're sick, and somebody needs to do something. Either get them training, protective gear or whatever they need so that they can work without being made sick...." And so the older guy [police officer] said, "Well, you know, you don't know where you are. And this is just how it is, and you better just do your job as a nurse and leave this alone." And he was very final in his tone. So I thought, well, I can't argue with this guy. Then they left. But then a few minutes later, the younger guy came back and he said, "I know what you're talking about." He said, "It's, it's wrong and he's right, it is how things are down here." He said, "But, you know, we appreciate anybody that wants to try to help, but it's a pretty well-established system."

—RN: Hurricane Katrina

"I Did What I Thought Was Best"

Although making everyday decisions can be difficult, in disaster/humanitarian response the difficulty is multiplied exponentially due to the surrounding chaos and uncertainty. Respondents struggle to make the *best* decision in consideration of the environment, scope of practice, available resources, and professional experience; however, seeking what is *best* may be a double-edge sword. Support to resolve questions of moral content is tenuous given the absence of an ethicist and the complexity of decision-making with chaplains who may provide guidance from within a religious framework. The sharp reality is that decisions can affect responders for the duration of deployment and thereafter.

> *The last thing you have time to do is pull out your 800-page manual and start leafing through it to find out what you're supposed to be doing.*
> —*Paramedic: Chemical Explosion*

> *It's an emotional toll. A man, regardless of how strong he is mentally, emotionally, and physically, can only bear so much weight for so long. And there's got to be a point where, you have to, you have to sit down with somebody, you have to talk to somebody, you have to get it off your chest. You can't continue to hold it in, or you're gonna be hit hard, you're gonna be tore apart. It all boils down to an emotional toll that it takes on your psyche as time goes on.*
> —*Fire/EMT: California wildfires*

> *If you think…"I'm making a decision," and try and think through it the way you would think through things in the real world, it may give you too many options. You're in these situations, and the resources are so limited, every kind of resource you can imagine. I mean that building with 2000 people in it for the first couple of days only had 2 restrooms for all those people. That's a resource limitation. You have limitations of supplies. You've got limitations on oxygen. You have limitations on who to talk to, to know what to do or to get things done. But when you have a moral conflict, there's no one to pick up and call for somebody to help you out there…[When seeking guidance from a chaplain] if everything sort of takes on a particular religious frame, that might or might not be helpful.*
> —*RN: Cambodian Refugee Crisis*

DISCUSSION

Responder stories are rich in their assertions that ethical compromise produces duress. Moral uncertainty is ubiquitous within disaster settings, and ethical boundaries are tested during reconciliation. Literature indicates that the extent to which responders apply ethical principles to decision-making is unknown.[7,8] This article demonstrates responders' awareness of ethical principles and moral behavior; however, moral versus immoral behavior presents a dichotomy to be reckoned with.[26] Consequently, disaster/humanitarian responders are susceptible to distress when moral boundaries are violated.

Although ethics terminology was not widely used, responders shared experiences in which they were cognizant of ethical principles, such as justice, beneficence, nonmaleficence, and respect for autonomy. Despite the challenges of chaotic settings, responders often face the risk of personal harm in their efforts to ensure the well-being of others. In this study, Western values and belief in the sanctity of life overrode a victim's desire to be released from life. Despite adherence to personal convictions of what was morally correct, and practicing in a way she believed to be right, internal conflict occurred as the responder questioned within herself if this was the choice that would typically have been made within the local culture. In reflection, the question about what was right for the patient endured.

A common, utilitarian goal is to ensure the best outcome for the greatest number of survivors through the most efficient use of available resources.[6] In the current study, although lack of resources resulted in moral compromise, responders shared stories of their ability to think critically when providing care with limited resources. One participant shared that responders "*McGyver*" resources, or improvise, using on-hand supplies when necessary to safeguard survivors' safety and security. Essential supplies are key to ensuring that responders have the critical items needed to accomplish tasks within chaotic disaster/humanitarian environments.

Understandably, when responders cannot fulfill their mission to restore a degree of normalcy to stricken individuals and communities, moral incongruence occurs. A lack of supplies constrains the ethical nature of the social contract between disaster/humanitarian responders and affected individuals and communities. Likewise, the lack of ability to perform ethically is a barrier to providing care in a manner that adheres to professional codes of conduct [for example, American Medical Association, American Nurses Association].

Literature does not address how limitations in time to respond affects responder mental health; however, Almonte[27] alludes to the concept of time and its impact on responder mental health when sharing that humanitarian nurses on the USNS *Mercy* experienced "anguish" (p. 483), and described their brief interval to provide care as "heartbreaking" and meager like applying a "mere bandaid." These findings are similar to the current study wherein responders' deployment was abbreviated, and long-term recovery of those they encountered was unknown. Similarly, the nurses in Almonte's[27] study expressed feelings of helplessness due to not being able to provide care as a result of lack of services.

Responders shared that having someone to confer with when making morally complex decisions would be helpful. Although volunteer chaplains may be available, one participant shared that support characterized by religious undertones may not be beneficial. This is likely due to the diversity of faith, spirituality, and cultural influences among responders. Literature does not address the beneficial presence of faith-based providers and other laypersons other than to allege that delays in their arrival to the disaster/humanitarian event may be more beneficial due to the amount of time needed for responder emotional and mental stress to manifest.[28]

Disaster/humanitarian settings are complex, and scenarios within them cannot be characterized as traditional. Additionally, the unexpected nature of disasters limits the ability to prepare for moral and emotional conflicts that are inherent in response.[27,28] Consequently, responders new to disaster/humanitarian efforts may require additional care to ensure mental health. Although seasoned responders may have developed coping mechanisms to overcome incapacitating emotional distress, attention also must be provided to ensure that these professionals do not succumb to incapacitating mental and physiologic sequelae of the response experience.

SUMMARY

This article has provided numerous avenues for additional research when exploring the impact of moral incongruence on disaster/humanitarian responders. Among them is exploration of optimal coping methods for responders given the unique characteristics of disaster/humanitarian settings, an examination of the mental health impact of moral decision-making processes when immersed in differing cultures, assessment of decision-making frameworks for use in austere settings, and investigation into the of feasibility of a "disaster ethicist" role so as to provide support for moral decision-making. Literature alludes to the need for ethical decision-making frameworks; however, there is no indication that the decision derived from use of a framework would eliminate responder distress. Rather, the framework would guide decision-making leaving potential distress derived from the decision to be dealt with. Mental health is but one component in retention of disaster/humanitarian responders whose knowledge, compassion, and concern for the well-being of others is vital to survival during this season of what many believe to be an increase in man-made and natural disasters.[29,30]

REFERENCES

1. Daniel M. Bedside resource stewardship in disasters: a provider's dilemma practicing in an ethical gap. J Clin Ethics 2012;23(4):331–5.
2. Peter E, Liaschenko J. Perils of proximity: a spatiotemporal analysis of moral distress and moral ambiguity. Nurs Inq 2004;11(4):218–25.
3. International Committee of the Red Cross [ICRC]. The code of conduct for the International Red Cross and Red Crescent Movement and Non-Governmental Organisations (NGOs) in disaster relief (n.d.). Available at: https://www.icrc.org/eng/assets/files/publications/icrc-002-1067.pdf. Accessed August 14, 2014.
4. American Nurses Association. Short definitions of ethical principles and theories familiar words, what do they mean? [n.d.]. Available at: http://www.nursingworld.org/MainMenuCategories/EthicsStandards/Resources/. Accessed April 22, 2016.
5. Health and Human Services [HHS]. The Belmont report. 1979. Available at: http://www.hhs.gov/ohrp/regulations-and-policy/belmont-report/index.html#xbenefit. Accessed April 22, 2016.
6. Wagner J, Dahnke M, Pomona NJ. Nursing ethic and disaster triage: applying utilitarian ethical theory. J Emerg Nurs 2015;41(4):300–6.
7. Hunt MR. Establishing moral bearings: ethics and expatriate health care professionals in humanitarian work. Disasters 2011;35(3):606–22.
8. Johnson K. The professionalization of the humanitarian role: ethics and accountability. Symposium conducted at the meeting of Medecins Sans Frontieres, Montreal, Canada, February 01, 2011.
9. Hunt MR. Moral experience of Canadian healthcare professionals in humanitarian work. Prehosp Disaster Med 2009;24(6):518–24.
10. Alexander DA, Klein S. First responders after disasters: a review of stress reactions, at-risk, vulnerability, and resilience factors. Prehosp Disaster Med 2009;24(2):87–94.
11. Meeker E, Plum K, Veenema T. Management of the psychosocial effects of disasters. In: Veenema TG, editor. Disaster nursing and emergency preparedness of chemical, biological, and radiological terrorism and other hazards. 3rd edition. New York: Springer; 2013. p. 111–30.
12. Lönnqvist JE, Walkowitz G, Wichardt P, et al. The moderating effect of conformism values on the relations between other personal values, social norms, moral obligation, and single altruistic behaviours. Br J Soc Psychol 2009;48(Pt 3):525–46.
13. Center for the Study of Traumatic Stress (CSTS). Sustaining caregiving and psychological well-being while caring for disaster victims. 2014. Available at: http://www.cstsonline:wp-content/resources/philippines-typhoon/CSTS_Sustaining%20Psychological%20Well%20Being%20of%20Caregivers%20in%20Disasters.pdf. Accessed August 14, 2014.
14. Hodge JG Jr, Hanfling D, Powell TP. Practical, ethical, and legal challenges underlying crisis standards of care. J Law Med Ethics 2013;41(Suppl 1):50–5.
15. Knebel AR, Sharpe VA, Danis M, et al. Informing the gestalt: an ethical framework for allocating scarce federal public health and medical resources to states during disasters. Disaster Med Public Health Prep 2014;8(1):79–88.

16. Institute of Medicine. Crisis standards of care: a systems framework for catastrophic disaster response, 2012 catastrophic disaster response. 2012. Available at: http://www.nap.edu/catalog/13351/crisis-standards-of-care-a-systems-framework-for-catastrophic-disaster. Accessed June 01, 2014.

17. Hunt MR, Sindling C, Schwartz L. Tragic choices in humanitarian health work. J Clin Ethics 2012;23(4):333–44.

18. Schwartz L. Does ethics travel? Symposium conducted at the meeting of Medecins Sans Frontieres, Montreal, Canada, February 01, 2011.

19. Hunt MR, Schwartz L, Fraser V. "How far do you go and where are the issues surrounding that?" Dilemmas at the boundaries of clinical competency in humanitarian health work. Prehosp Disaster Med 2013;28(5):502–8.

20. Slim H. Doing the right thing: relief agencies, moral dilemmas and responsibility in political emergencies and war. Disasters 1997;21(3):244–57.

21. Corley MC. Nurse moral distress: a proposed theory and research agenda. Nurs Ethics 2002;9(6):636–50.

22. Nash WP, Marino Carper TL, Mills MA, et al. Psychometric evaluation of the moral injury events scale. Mil Med 2013;178(6):646–52.

23. Johnstone MJ, Hutchinson A. 'Moral distress' – time to abandon a flawed nursing construct? Nurs Ethics 2015;22(1):5–14.

24. Boswell S. "I saved the iguana": a mixed methods study examining responder mental health after major disasters and humanitarian relief events [dissertation]. Knoxville (TN): University of Tennessee; 2014.

25. Thomas S, Pollio H. Listening to patients: a phenomenological approach to nursing research and practice. New York: Springer Publishing; 2002.

26. Lofquist L. Virtues and humanitarian ethics. Disasters 2016. [Epub ahead of print].

27. Almonte A. Humanitarian nursing challenges: a grounded theory study. Mil Med 2009;174(5):479–85.

28. Stone A. Beyond debriefing: how to address responder's emotional health. Emergency Management; 2013. Available at: http://www.emergencymgmt.com/training/Beyond-Debriefing-Responders-Emotional-Health.html?page=2.

29. ReliefWeb. Global increase in climate related disasters. 2015. Available at: http://reliefweb.int/sites/reliefweb.int/files/resources/global-increase-climate-related-disasters.pdf. Accessed April 22, 2016.

30. Forsyth A, Smeade L. Health and places initiative. Disasters, health, and place. A research brief. Version 1.0. 2014. Available at: http://research.gsd.harvard.edu/hapi/. Accessed April 22, 2016.

Federal Emergency Management Agency Response in Rural Appalachia

A Tale of Miscommunication, Unrealistic Expectations, and "Hurt, Hurt, Hurt"

Lauren M. Oppizzi, MSN, RN[a], Susan Speraw, PhD, RN[b],*

KEYWORDS

- Federal Emergency Management Agency (FEMA) • Disaster
- Emergency management • Rural • Appalachia • Phenomenology
- Interprofessional collaboration • Policy

KEY POINTS

- Rural residents often lack understanding of rules pertaining to disaster declarations and eligibility for federal disaster assistance; this includes misunderstanding of the roles of Federal Emergency Management Agency (FEMA) inspectors.
- Poverty, geographic isolation, and low resource availability magnify disaster vulnerability in rural areas.
- Nurses, as trusted community members, are in a position to be effective advocates for survivors, working in interprofessional collaborative practice with local officials to explain in jargon-free language the specifics of governmental rules, expectations, and the process of applying for federal aid.
- Including rural residents in disaster research is part of the social contract between government and citizens; rural voices should have weight equal to urban perspectives in informing public policy.
- Criteria for determining disaster aid eligibility should be reappraised, adjusted downward for high-poverty areas where it is difficult to meet the current federal standard for damages.

Disclosure: See last page of article.
[a] University of Tennessee College of Nursing, Knoxville, 1200 Volunteer Boulevard, Knoxville, TN 37396, USA; [b] University of Tennessee College of Nursing, Knoxville, Signal Mountain, TN 37377, USA
* Corresponding author.
E-mail address: ssperaw@utk.edu

Nurs Clin N Am 51 (2016) 599–611
http://dx.doi.org/10.1016/j.cnur.2016.07.012
0029-6465/16/© 2016 Elsevier Inc. All rights reserved.

INTRODUCTION

The state of Kentucky reflects 2 extreme poles of reality. Northern metropolitan areas consolidate wealth and distinction. In contrast, sparsely populated southeastern mountain communities experience struggle and poverty equal to that of developing nations.[1] Scarred by mine closures and job loss, hampered by poor health and low educational attainment, rural towns have endured population decline and seen prospects for growth stifled by the absence of reliable infrastructure and basic services.[2–8] Nevertheless, southeastern Kentucky is also a place that binds people together with a powerful sense of "being home" among the deeply rutted dirt roads leading into hollows that shelter entire families. Traditions and oral history give residents an intimate connection to each other and to land that has for generations welcomed each new life and cradled the ashes of their dead. Here, trust in God runs deep; relationships form the bedrock of community, and the most valuable currency is one's word.[9,10] Against this complex backdrop, disaster management takes place (**Fig. 1**).

Rural preparedness has been identified as a national vulnerability since 2002.[11] Disproportionate shares of responsibility for community well-being fall on rural hospitals and health centers, despite the reality that these entities have fewer resources, a greater geographic area to serve, and far less surge capacity than is found in larger cities.[12,13] Aged, crumbling infrastructure also increases susceptibility to a host of natural disasters. All of these challenges impact preparedness in southeastern Kentucky.

Floods are the state's greatest natural disaster risk, with most frequent declared events occurring in the southeast.[14–16] Since 1978, state residents have received hundreds of millions of dollars in flood insurance payouts following torrential rains,[14] yet with nearly 40% of residents in southeastern counties living in poverty,[4–7] few actually hold flood insurance. The remainder relies on the compassion of charitable organizations; federal aid is reserved for the few residing in areas declared eligible. In 2012, Federal Emergency Management Agency (FEMA) payouts of more than $18.6 million were distributed among just 23 of Kentucky's 120 counties, even though residents of many other counties also lost everything.[17] Hidden costs of disaster add additional burden, including those resulting from exposure to toxins, mold, or infectious diseases that come in the wake of flooding.[18]

Among the general population, there is little understanding of how FEMA determines eligibility for disaster assistance. The assumption is that FEMA aid is generous and easy to obtain, when in fact the opposite is true.[19,20] Following disaster, a well-choreographed process takes place through which state governors first activate their state emergency plan; determine that the required response is beyond the financial capacity of their jurisdiction; and subsequently request, via the Secretary of Homeland Security, a Presidential declaration. Initial damage assessments, conducted by FEMA agents working with local officials, result in a determination whether to recommend to the President that a declaration be issued. Damage assessments are based on a single, per capita figure, currently $1.35; this means that in a state with 10 million people, computed eligible damage estimates would need to reach $13.5 million before a presidential declaration would be issued.[21] This figure may be attainable in high-population areas, but in rural communities where poverty is high and property values are low, reaching this figure can be problematic. Indeed, most requests for FEMA aid are denied because damage is insufficient to meet the standard.[20] Although this process and its limitations are clear to government officials, local residents may not realize that FEMA agents on their property may not assure aid. When victims confront the reality of losing everything, the logic and fairness of FEMA determinations often generate

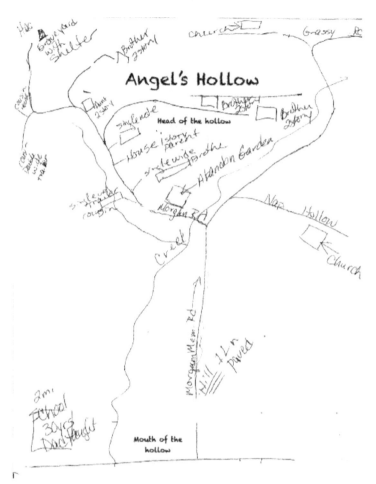

Fig. 1. "Angel's Hollow" was drawn by a local resident: her own Appalachian hollow. It illustrates ways in which kinship networks live in proximity, in conventional houses (1- or 2-story) and trailers (single or double-wide), near a family cemetery and church. Closeness provides both mutual security and sources of material assistance. With only one road, hollows increase disaster vulnerability: difficult to reach and treacherous or impossible to escape.

anger or confusion.[19] Mitigating the psychological consequences of denied federal aid becomes an important question for communities.

Recent trends in health care, which favor interprofessional collaborative practice, are in keeping with practice recommendations in rural health.[13,22] Incorporating the input of all community members makes information sharing more effective, and having "all hands on deck" regardless of professional discipline or citizens' roles in the community enables support to be given when and how it is needed most. Collaboration provides vital linkages between rural communities and government agencies; most importantly, it creates synergy to maintain critical infrastructure.[23] Nurses, often the most trusted people in communities, can be of assistance not only in providing direct health services or helping in rescue and rebuilding efforts but also in interprofessional collaboration to educate local residents about how and when to apply for aid, interpret government jargon, and reduce disasters' negative impact on health (**Fig. 2**).[23]

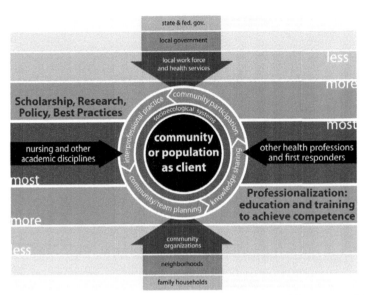

Fig. 2. Interprofessional collaborative practice in disaster: nurses working as part of interprofessional teams play a role in working with the community as client, engaged with other disciplines, and citizens in a process of information sharing and planning. (*Courtesy of* Susan Speraw, PhD, RN; Moriah McArthur, MSc; Joleen Darragh, M. Arch; 2011.)

This qualitative research aimed to describe the experiences of rural Appalachian residents who, in 2012, interfaced with FEMA inspectors after flooding that resulted in a presidentially declared disaster for 23 counties.

METHODS

Following University of Tennessee, Knoxville Institutional Review Board approval, 9 English-speaking residents of southeastern Kentucky were recruited as participants in the study. All met 5 inclusion criteria: (a) 18 years old or older; (b) resident of southeastern Kentucky; (c) affected by the floods of 2012; (d) participated in a preliminary damage assessment by FEMA; and (e) willing to participate in a recorded phenomenological interview. Recruitment occurred (a) through mailings announcing the study sent to impacted residents by the Director of Emergency Management; this was the individual who facilitated the original contact between community members and FEMA following the flooding of 2012; (b) flyers posted at a community outreach center; and (c) word of mouth. Before conducting the study, the investigators were known to community leaders as a result of their work on the federally funded Appalachia Community Health and Disaster Readiness Project; relationships with trusted community leaders facilitated the success of the study.

Interviews, which ranged from 30 to 60 minutes, were digitally recorded, transcribed verbatim, and analyzed using a phenomenological approach according to Thomas and Pollio.[24] Interviews focused on the process of discovering "the immediacy of human experience from the expert perspective of the one who lives it."[24] Because of poverty, low literacy, and geographic isolation, Appalachian community members often live unseen and unheard at the margins of power in society. The phenomenological approach was selected because it is appropriate where cultural factors play a critical role in mediating relationships, and because it respects each person's experience of reality, allowing their voice to be heard.

Face-to-face interviews were conducted by the principal investigator at a private location that was mutually agreeable. After obtaining informed consent, the investigator led the interview with the question, "When you think about your experience after the flood of 2012, what stands out for you about the process of applying for assistance from FEMA?" There was no survey or set schedule of questions. The interview continued until the participant exhausted the topic and their narration of experience. Each participant received a $20 gift card to compensate for time and gas money.

RESULTS

Nine participants were interviewed, with ages ranging from the 40s into the 70s. In this article, they are identified with pseudonyms. Their homes reflected the full spectrum of housing in rural Appalachia: trailers and conventional homes constructed with brick, wood, and cement block. All participants lost much or all of their housing and possessions, yet none of them lived in counties declared eligible for federal assistance (**Table 1**).

CONTEXTUAL GROUND OF EXPERIENCE: THE STORM

By all accounts, the storm arrived with fury and power that was immediate:

My husband didn't expect rain like that...but then, here come an entire big metal building, twelve by twenty-four feet...and everything in it [floating by], the water was so high...rough. He said water rushed in and that building just went right across the driveway and down the creek.

—Jenny

Participants began their narratives by detailing the way the flooding impacted their psychological and physical well-being. Tammy told how floodwaters rushed into her home:

It was scary...there was no way out... I was going to use the bathroom and by the time I got [finished] the water was almost to our knees...and I said, "Please turn

Table 1
Participants' homes reflected the full range of housing in rural Appalachia: despite the fact that all participants lost much or all of their housing and possessions, they lived in counties declared ineligible for assistance, leaving them with few avenues for help

Pseudonym	Gender	Age Range	Type of Residential Construction	Was County of Residence Eligible for FEMA Assistance?
Tammy	Female	40s	Cement block	No
Kelsey	Female	50s	Brick	No
Thomas	Male	50s	Brick	No
Betsy	Female	60s	Wood	No
Joanne	Female	50s	Brick	No
Joe	Male	50s	Brick	No
Jenny	Female	50s	Wood	No
Bill	Male	70s	Trailer	No
Marilyn	Female	70s	Trailer	No

that [electrical] breaker off.".... That's all I could think about. They said that if I didn't [shut down the power], electricity would have killed us all... I sat my grand-baby in the window sill, it was so bad. He was wanting to play in [the flood water] and I said, "No, baby. It's not water to play in." ...The tile and shoes from our closets was floating through our house... we never thought we was going to get out alive... All I could say was, "Lord, please let the water go down. Don't let it get no higher." Because we knew if the water went down we would be fine. But standing there in water we were saying, "Please Lord, help us."... If He wouldn't have been there... I would have never got through what I got through.

KEY ELEMENTS OF THE FEDERAL EMERGENCY MANAGEMENT AGENCY EXPERIENCE
"All We Lost"

After describing the storm, participants typically recapped all they lost in the flood: gravel roads, barns, livestock, hay feeders, fencing, bridges, furniture, flooring, vehicles, mowers, homes, land, their hard-earned livelihoods and security, and mental well-being. Tammy summed her experience, "We had nothing left. We had to start completely all over again."

From participants' perspectives, FEMA did not connect with the magnitude and reality of what was washed away. Residents believed that damage determination should not have been merely an exercise in estimating the value of a new ceiling. What residents also wanted FEMA workers to understand was what the lost or damaged items represented in their lives. When possessions washed away, participants lost property that had been in their family for generations. When cows drowned, residents lost income and a way to provide food for their families. When fences were ripped down by floodwaters, the security of their land was lost. Worst of all, because of poverty, there was no way to replace things that were swept away.

[Floods] took everything we had.... [FEMA agent] wrote down the house damage, but he wasn't writing anything down about the cow, the fence, and the stuff we lost.

—Kelsey

"Hurt, Hurt, Hurt"

Hurt described the emotional impact of both the flood and the interactions with FEMA. The sudden loss of property and homes was overwhelming. Two years after the flood, Bill, an elderly resident of the area, is still unable to sleep, haunted by memories of losing his animals and hearing them "screaming" as floodwaters swept them away. He recalled his "terrible...horrible...scariest" experience as his daughter nearly died: "Our daughter about drowned...she went under and [our son] had to pick her up by the hair of the head, and drag her up over the water.... [since then] I don't sleep none in the night." Thomas tearfully recounted his experience, describing how he had thought, "the end of time is coming."

Although the flood was traumatic, it was clear that FEMA representatives were the great antagonists in each participant story. FEMA agents stepped onto the scene after the flood and, with words and actions, disrespected residents; lack of communication and failure to explain their process resulted in false hope. Betsy described her experience: "FEMA called me to let me know they were coming... We waited a whole day; we didn't go anywhere. Nobody showed up." In other instances, FEMA agents inspected homes and property, stated outright or implied they would be back to help, and never returned. Joe tearfully shared his disappointment, concluding, "the worst hurt is, I got fooled [by FEMA]." When discussing whether she would rely on FEMA if another disaster were to befall her, Tammy replied, "To be honest with you, probably not... because [what they did] really hurts."

Interactions between residents and FEMA personnel caused hurt that cut to the core of participants' perceived value as human beings.

> People that's got fancy homes, they can get what they want done. They've got their roads back, tunnels put back in. We poor people got nothing.
>
> —Tammy

Time and again, residents' comments reflected the belief that if someone was marginalized and poor, FEMA had no interest in helping them.

> The poor man gets nothing....he's the last one they check on.
>
> —Bill

Reverberating loudly in the responses of all participants was the sense of having been devalued through interactions with FEMA. Residents felt written off from the start.

"There Was Not Enough Damage"

Related to hurt and devaluation was the feeling of having been betrayed by government agents who were supposedly committed to helping. In at least one circumstance, a family was told that their trailer was condemned based on the preliminary assessment. FEMA assessors suggested that the family leave the home untouched and stay temporarily with a friend or relative until FEMA could deliver a trailer to replace their home. When they eventually learned no help would be coming, the family's only recourse was to do what they could to salvage what remained. Nevertheless, on their return to their property, they found that during the delay structural damage had worsened:

> FEMA said they would probably help us get a trailer but they never done nothing to help. They come back and said we didn't have enough damage. I mean my house was damaged. Everything in it was destroyed... [Eventually] we just went [back] and we started cleaning everything up... You know, we could have took our furniture out to begin with instead [of listening to FEMA] telling us to wait. Where the mold was in [the walls] and FEMA said, "Just leave it alone," we took every bit of that out...put new walls, and finally everything washed down with bleach and every bit of the mold out before we went in there [to live] because mold can kill you.
>
> —Tammy

People in the community knew how Tammy's family was treated, and many participants referenced it in their interviews. FEMA's failure to help someone who had so clearly sustained massive damage contributed to the community's sense of hopelessness and betrayal. Thomas commented, "If FEMA ain't going to help (Tammy) when the water went square through the house and they had to take a boat and go out there and get them out, then [FEMA] ain't going to do nothing for me."

Several weeks after FEMA agents made their evaluations, residents heard about the decision that there was not enough damage to warrant federal assistance.

> FEMA is just...not a person to count on. They will tell you one thing and do another. It really hurt because you lose everything and they say, "Well, we might get you this...just hold on and let us do what we've gotta do." And then FEMA

come back and say, "No. There's nothing we can do. We can't even help you with nothing."

—Joanne

"That's the Trouble…Lack of Communication"

Misunderstandings about FEMA were universal. Even the most polite comments about FEMA were disparaging, with agents described as unresponsive, uncaring, and, at their worst, dishonest. Joe observed, "There was a write-up in the [local newspaper] of how much money was coming into the county for repairs and to help flood victims, but somebody must have stuck that money in their pocket because we never did see anything."

Without fail, everybody talked about FEMA as a nameless, faceless entity that was detached and made no connection with the community. Inspectors came into participants' homes, took pictures, and wrote things down, but they offered no identification, no explanation of what they were doing, no guidance about what to anticipate, and no instructions for when or how to apply for federal aid.

I knew somebody was coming, and if it wasn't for the mark on the car I wouldn't have known who it was…they didn't even introduce themselves.

—Betsy

Only one participant made statements that indicated she had basic understanding of how FEMA worked and that there was a financial threshold of damages that needed to be reached before federal aid would be available. Having that little bit of knowledge helped temper her expectations and disappointment:

FEMA done what they could…there's got to be a certain amount [of damage]… there's got to be a lot of people that had lost homes before FEMA could help [us] put everything back [to the way it was].

—Jenny

Other respondents were like Betsy, a woman who explained that her expectations were based on what she saw on television: "When you see [FEMA] on TV or hear about it, they're supposed to be helping people… I was expecting they would do more than they did." Other expectations were based on promises given by representatives that they would or might return with help. What residents actually experienced contrasted with these promises, yielding frustration and powerlessness:

They didn't communicate with us. More or less all they done was come in our house and said, "It's a disaster…everything's destroyed…let everything go. We will come back once we make a decision." There's nobody higher than FEMA, so why would you argue with them?

—Tammy

Lack of communication, follow-up, and aid undermined pre-existing public confidence in emergency management organizations. One resident offered the important observation that victims were unaware of how to reach FEMA or apply for federal aid:

[The FEMA representative] said, "There has been a lot of water under your house." I said, "Yeah. I knew that." And he said, "We will be back." He wrote my name down and I never did see him no more… I never did contact them. I didn't really know <u>how</u> to contact them.

—Thomas

Participants' disparaging descriptions of FEMA stood in stark contrast to positive qualities attributed to local sources of help. FEMA may have more money and resources, but it was representatives from local agencies—the director of the hospital, church pastors, and school principals—who communicated, introduced themselves, provided water, and were faithful to their word. FEMA representatives had powerful credentials, but in terms of commitment and fidelity to their mission, they fell far short in participants' estimation:

Nobody knows how [they] are gonna have the money to put [their house] back together. And then somebody like [the church mission] comes along and helps you, and that's wonderful, for someone to take from their church's donations and help us when no one else would… [The mission] is not like [FEMA] that says, "Yeah, we will be back. We will do this; we will do that." [but don't]… [the people at the mission] are higher than FEMA ever thought about being… I'm thanking God you've got somebody out there in the world like that, because if you didn't [poor people] wouldn't have no one.

—Tammy

"We at Least Had Hope"

When asked how it felt when FEMA said they would return, Marilyn described her immediate thoughts: "We had hope!" Sadly, the hope that FEMA generated through their presence in the community, interactions with residents, property damage surveys, and the confidence in government that FEMA embodied were all short-lived.

As it became evident that FEMA would not be a source of hoped-for assistance, people were left with the bedrock beliefs that had sustained them through the flood and its aftermath: their belief in the providence of God.

God has took care of [us] this long, He'll finish it out.

—Bill

… the Lord showed me, "I'll restore back to you." So far all I'm lacking is my fence and my lawnmower… I know He don't have nothing to do with these material things, but He gives us strength where we can work and have it.

—Jenny

Loss of material objects was a great source of disappointment, but interviewees did not let this undermine their hope or ability to press on through hardship. Although grieving for all they had lost, they set to work to rebuild with thankfulness in their hearts and the belief that God orchestrated all circumstances:

You can always get these little material things back. I know it's God's work. He gives and He takes. So just be thankful.

—Jenny

At the time of the interviews, 2 years after the disaster, all of the participants were still living in the homes that were flooded. Some residences had remnants of significant damage and were affected by mold, which had a negative impact on health. However, "day by day" their diligence paid off and homes were on the path to restoration.

…we went ahead and put the garden back out…and now I've got tomatoes and potatoes. They've done real good this year. And so it's getting back.

—Jenny

Despite their experience with FEMA, hope endures.

What we're living on is hope. Hope for a better day.

—Bill

DISCUSSION

Findings from this research validate the unique vulnerabilities of rural populations and illustrate the complex dilemmas that face government representatives and health care providers responding to disasters in isolated or rural communities. Narratives and the themes that they generated have implications for policy, practice, and future research.

Implications for Policy

Participants' comments illustrate that there is much work to be done to optimize effectiveness of federal representatives. Joanne's reference to FEMA as not a "person to count on" illustrates a fundamental misunderstanding of the distinction between an impersonal government agency functioning on strict criteria, and charitable local agencies whose mission it is to flex, responding to local need by lending a saving hand. Thomas and Joe were unaware of how to apply for federal aid. Given that destruction of property was so complete, community members could not conceive that no help would be forthcoming. Common sense said that if the totality of one's house and possessions was washed away, no one would dispute that there was "enough" damage. By coming onto residents' property without explaining their purposes or the limits of their obligation, FEMA agents entered into what residents perceived as an implied contract, and like any contractor, those agents would be held to account and expected to return to do the needed work. Instead, most residents never heard directly from FEMA again and were left to learn through word of mouth that no help would be forthcoming. Those that did receive word were told that losing everything was "not enough." Residents felt marginalized because they were poor, abandoned by their government, and denied services accorded to people of higher socioeconomic status. Remedies for these ills are not impossible to craft. Simple measures, such as having FEMA inspectors keep appointments and honor people's time; introduce themselves by name; provide clear, nontechnical explanations about limits of aid, what residents can expect from the inspection, and specifics about how and when to apply for assistance, could go a long way toward forestalling misunderstandings and hurt. Public information ads free of jargon, placed on television and radio, could explain FEMA's process and how to apply for aid. Modifying the standard for determining property loss in poor, rural areas could help qualify more people for disaster assistance. Encounters with government should not leave citizens feeling they are less valued because of poverty or the remoteness of the place where they live and work.

Implications for Practice

With interprofessional and collaboration as the contemporary watchwords for clinical practice, health providers in rural communities are poised as never before to work in partnership with local officials, FEMA agents, and other disaster responders. Nurses, often the most trusted members of the community, through their training and experience are skilled in translating and interpreting technical jargon. As liaisons between government agents and local residents, they could smooth rough edges of surly inspectors, clarify expectations, and assist residents who qualify in applying for federal aid. Acting in this way, nurses could be effective agents in helping residents obtain maximum material assistance and reduce emotional stress associated with devastation and loss. While working with government inspectors, nurses could also simultaneously use the full range of their skills to assess the physical and emotional well-being of residents traumatized and exposed to infectious agents and hazards associated with disaster.

Implications for Research

Including rural populations in health care research cannot be optional. Even when population density is low and reaching residents is challenging, justice dictates that the voices of rural citizens must be heard and their perceptions considered in policy making. Evaluating rural communities after disaster is part of the social contract that governments—local, state, and federal—have with their citizens. Researching the experience of FEMA agents in rural areas could also highlight areas they identify as needs for further training.

DISCLAIMER

This research was completed during the time when the authors were involved in a public health project in the southeastern Kentucky region as part of the Appalachia Community Health and Disaster Readiness Interprofessional Collaborative Practice, Health Resources and Service Administration Grant No. UD7HP26205. This research was not part of the grant-funded project, however, and the findings and conclusions reported here do not necessarily reflect the views or opinions of the US Department of Health and Human Services or the Health Resources and Services Administration.

CONFLICT OF INTEREST

There are no conflicts of interest to report.

REFERENCES

1. Lowry A. What's the matter with Eastern Kentucky? New York Times Magazine 2014. Available at: http://www.nytimes.com/2014/06/29/magazine/whats-the-matter-with-eastern-kentucky-html. Accessed June 30, 2014.
2. Flippen A. Where are the hardest places to live in the U.S.? New York Times 2014. Available at: http://www.nytimes.com/2014/06/26/upshot/where-are-the-hardest-places-to-live-in-the-us.html. Accessed June 30, 2014.
3. U.S. Department of Health and Human Services, Health Resources and Services Administration, Health Professional Shortage Areas as of 04/07/2016—Kentucky. Available at: http://datawarehouse.hrsa.gov/tools/analyzers/HpsaFindResults.aspx. Accessed April 7, 2016.
4. The Foundation for a Healthy Kentucky. Data Source: Kentucky Department for Public Health (KDPH). Cumberland Valley Area Development District. Frankfort (KY): Cabinet for Health and Family Services; 2016.
5. The Foundation for a Healthy Kentucky. Data Source: Kentucky Department for Public Health (KDPH). Lake Cumberland Area Development District. Frankfort (KY): Cabinet for Health and Family Services; 2016.
6. The Foundation for a Healthy Kentucky. Data Source: Kentucky Department for Public Health (KDPH). Kentucky River Area Development District. Frankfort (KY): Cabinet for Health and Family Services; 2016.

7. The Foundation for a Healthy Kentucky. Data Source: Kentucky Department for Public Health (KDPH). Big Sandy Area Development District. Frankfort (KY): Cabinet for Health and Family Services; 2016.

8. Kentucky Department for Public Health, Cabinet for Health and Family Services. State health assessment: a compilation on health status. Frankfort (KY): Kentucky Department for Public Health; 2013.

9. Murray K. Down to earth people of Appalachia. Boone (NC): Appalachian Consortium Press; 1981.

10. Billings DB, Norman G, Ledford K. Back talk from Appalachia: confronting stereotypes. Lexington (KY): University of Kentucky Press; 2000.

11. Office of Rural Health Policy, Health Resources and Services Administration. Rural communities and emergency preparedness. Washington, DC: U.S. Department of Health and Human Services; 2002.

12. Putzer GJ, Koro-Ljungberg M, Duncan P. Critical challenges and impediments affecting rural physicians during a public health emergency. Disaster Med Public Health Prep 2012;6:342–8.

13. Grant Makers in Health. Rural health care: innovations in policy and practice (Issue Brief No. 34). Washington, DC: Grant Makers in Health; 2009.

14. Commonwealth of Kentucky. Floodplain management in Kentucky: quick guide. Frankfort (KY): Kentucky Division of Water/Flood Mitigation Program; 2009.

15. Kentucky Division of Emergency Management. Kentucky State enhanced hazard mitigation plan. Frankfort (KY): Commonwealth of Kentucky; 2010.

16. Center for Hazards Research and Policy Development, University of Kentucky Hazard Mitigation Plan. Louisville (KY): Center for Hazards Research and Policy; 2010.

17. FEMA. Federal disaster aid in Kentucky tops $18 million. Washington, DC: Federal Emergency Management Agency; 2012. Available at: www.fema.gov. Accessed April 3, 2016.

18. Azuma K, Ikeda K, Kagi N, et al. Effects of water-damaged homes after flooding: health status of the residents and the environmental risk factors. Int J Environ Health Res 2014;24(2):158–75. Available at: http://dx.doi.org.proxy.lib.utk.edu:90/10.1080/09603123.2013.800964. Accessed April 15, 2016.

19. Kousky C, Shabman L. The realities of federal disaster aid: the case of floods. Resources for the Future Issue Brief 2012;12-02:16.

20. Kousky C. Facts about FEMA household disaster aid: examining the 2008 floods and tornadoes in Missouri. Weather Clim Soc 2013;5:332–44. Available at: http://journals.ametsoc.org/doi/abs/10.1175/WCAS-D-12-00059.1. Accessed March 20, 2016.

21. United States Government Accountability Office (GAO). Federal disaster assistance: improved criteria needed to assess a jurisdiction's capability to respond and recover on its own. Washington, DC: GAO; 2012. Available at: www.gao.gov/assets/650/648162.pdf. Accessed April 15, 2016.

22. World Health Organization (WHO). Framework for action on interprofessional education and collaborative practice. Geneva (Switzerland): World Health Organization; 2010. Available at: www.who.int/hrh/.../framework_action/en/. Accessed December 30, 2011.

23. Speraw S. Offering a comprehensive curriculum for a graduate degree in disaster nursing. In: Stanley SR, Wolanski TA, editors. Designing and integrating a disaster preparedness curriculum: readying nurses for the [0]Please provide the professional degrees, city name for all the authors present in the source

line of Fig. 2.worst. Indianapolis (IN): Sigma Theta Tau International; 2015. p. 205–54.

24. Thomas S, Pollio H. Listening to patients: a phenomenological approach to nursing research and practice. New York: Springer Publishing Company, Inc; 2002.

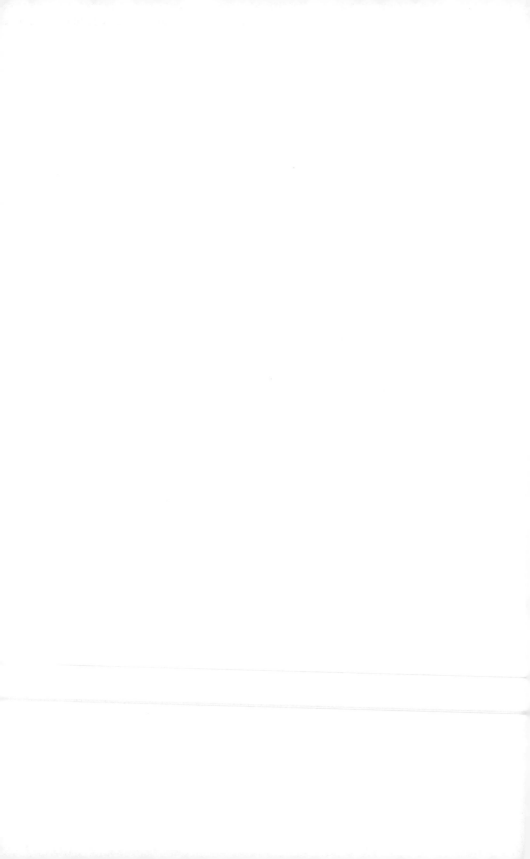

US Military Nurses
Serving Within the Chaos of Disaster

Felecia M. Rivers, PhD, RN[a,b],*

KEYWORDS

- Disaster response • Emotional response • Unknown • Existential growth
- Military nurses • Phenomenology

KEY POINTS

- Responding to disasters is not the same as going to combat. In war, you know what is expected. Going into a disaster, you are moving into the unknown.
- In war, you are prepared; plans are in place; basic systems are established. In disasters, you make do with what you have and use your ingenuity.
- Military members are expected to be strong and demonstrate endurance. However, during disaster response, their resiliency storehouses diminish. Nurses remarked that emotional issues may arise and linger.
- Disaster response changes an individual's perception of destruction. This new insight led to a greater appreciation of life.

INTRODUCTION

When you hear the word *disaster*, what thoughts or images come to mind? Do you picture a particular event you remember reading about or perhaps one broadcasted on the evening news? For military nurses who participated in this study, the word *disaster* has a very personal meaning because it is something they endured, an experience that will always stimulate special memories.

Disasters have been defined as "an event concentrated in time and space, in which a society … undergoes physical harm and social disruption".[1] Millions of individuals

Funding Sources: TriService Nursing Research Program (HU0001-08-1-TS16; N08-P12); Sigma Theta Tau International Honor Society of Nursing, Gamma Chi Chapter.
Disclaimer: This research was sponsored by the TriService Nursing Research Program, Uniformed Services University of the Health Sciences; however, the information or content and conclusions do not necessarily represent the official position or policy of, nor should any official endorsement be inferred by, the TriService Nursing Research Program, Uniformed Services of the Health Sciences. The views expressed herein are those of the author and do not reflect the official policy of the Department of the Army, Department of Defense, or the US government.
[a] Disaster Preparedness Emergency Management, Army Nurse Corps, PO Box 910, USA;
[b] Arkansas State University, Jonesboro, AR 72467, USA
* 6909 Ruggles Ferry Pike, Knoxville, TN 37924.
E-mail address: feleciarivers59@gmail.com

around the world fall subject to these catastrophic events each year. Moreover, the frequency and intensity of these events continue to increase. During these chaotic times, when the local disaster response efforts become overwhelmed, military forces may be requested to assist. The revised 2004 Stafford Act provides authorization for military units to be deployed for disaster response efforts that may include logistics, surveillance, sanitation, and medical support.[2] Since these acts have been written, federal health care providers, specifically military nurses, have increasingly been present during domestic and international disaster events to render care to those injured.

Historical nursing disaster response efforts began with the works of Florence Nightingale during the Crimean War, Jean-Henry Dunant's 1859 responses during the War of Italian Unification that lead to the establishment of the International Red Cross, and aid provided by Clara Barton in 1881 during the American Civil War, which resulted in the founding of the American Red Cross.[3,4] Continuing in 1923, military nurses began what has become an ongoing record of providing care during domestic and international incidents. That year, 2 groups of Army nurses provided disaster relief following an earthquake that destroyed a city in the Philippines. In the 1960s, military nurses responded to Chile, Iran, Alaska, and Yugoslavia after earthquakes and tidal waves to render aid. Responding in the early 1970s, military nurses provided assistance during a Nicaraguan earthquake and supported Operation New Life and New Arrivals involving Indochinese refugees into the United States after the Vietnam War.[5]

In more recent times, thousands of military nurses have continued to be instrumental in both domestic and international disaster responses. Some of these efforts include the 1992 famine crisis in Somalia, the 2004 Banda Aceh tsunami, Hurricane Katrina, the earthquake in Pakistan, the 2010 earthquakes in Haiti, Japan's 2012 earthquake and tsunami, and, in 2013, Hurricane Sandy. However, the number of nurses who have participated in disasters is poorly documented.[6–13]

The preponderance of existing published research focuses on military nurses' experiences in combat, but little is known about these nurses' experiences in disaster response and how to better provide for their well-being.

Therefore, the purpose of this study was to gain an understanding of the essence of military nurses' experiences in responding to disasters. One research question drove the study: What is the experience of military nurses during and/or following a disaster response? For this study, *disaster* was defined as any noncombat mission, such as humanitarian relief or response to a natural or human-made event outside of warfare.

The military nurses who participated in this study began to fill the gap in scientific knowledge through their stories. As a result, we have a better understanding of what disaster response entails, told to us through the voice of the experts. The outcomes of this research adds to the practical information regarding the overwhelming effects, response actions, readiness, and training needs of military nurses who have responded to disasters in the past. The findings can help us better prepare to assist those who may respond to these traumatic events in the future.

METHODS

A qualitative method was used to illuminate the nurses' experiences in responding to disasters. Existential phenomenology founded on Merleau-Ponty's philosophy, as described by Thomas and Pollio,[14] was used to conduct the research. This method allows the participant to provide data through their words based on experiences as they lived them; their voices become personified and alive as their stories unfold. A purposeful, snowball sampling method was used to elicit participants.

ETHICAL CONSIDERATION

An Institutional Review Board approved the study. During the study, pseudonyms were given to each person that volunteered. Those pseudonyms did not match the initials of either their first or last name.

SAMPLE

US military nurses from all service branches to include reservists and US Public Health Service Nurses who had responded to at least one disaster were invited to participate in the study. It was not known how many nurses in the targeted population fit the criteria of the study. The invitation to participate began with 2 nurses known to the principal investigator who had assisted in disaster response. They were requested to share study information with others who met the study criteria. Additionally, the invitation was e-mailed to military nurses from different branches known to the principal investigator. They were asked to distribute the information to their nurse colleagues within their perspective branches. No limit was placed on time from disaster response to volunteering for the interview or the type of disaster event (natural or man-made). Twenty-three nurses volunteered for the study. Saturation was obtained.

PROCEDURE

Following the consent process, open-ended, unstructured, single, face-to-face interviews were conducted at a time and place of the participant's choice. The different places selected included offices, participant homes, or conference rooms. Every interview began with a single question: *When you think about your disaster deployment, what stands out for you?* Probe questions were asked for clarification of previously mentioned information and to encourage description of their experiences. Interviews lasted from 27 to 90 minutes depending on the amount of information shared and concluded when each participant indicated they had nothing left to say. Each session was digitally recorded and transcribed by a professional transcriptionist, and the primary investigator validated the transcripts.

DATA ANALYSIS

Line-by-line analysis that identified key words and phrases within and across all transcripts led to the formulation of themes that emerged. This information was shared with the research team for discussion and validation. Once this was accomplished, a thematic structure, supported by verbatim texts, was developed. To ensure the data were interpreted accurately, member checking was conducted. A summary of the study along with the thematic structure was shared with the research participants following data analysis. One individual's comment was particularly poignant:

> I read your findings ... I literally had to stop several times because I had tears flowing. You captured the concrete and the inferred and placed an analysis of my thoughts/feelings that I was unable to put into words myself...you and your research have had a significant impact on my healing ... [It] let me know I am ok, I am normal ... we are all someplace between joy and pain.

RESULTS

The nurses responded to different types of calamitous events, including natural and man-made disasters that occurred between 1989 and 2008. These traumatic occurrences involved hurricanes, floods, tornadoes, earthquakes, plane crashes, flu epidemics, and terrorism-related incidences. Of the response actions, 13 were domestic and 9 were international. **Table 1** depicts the participants' demographic characteristics. **Table 2** provides a list of the different disasters and dates of response.

SHARING OF THE NARRATIVES

It should be noted that the length of time from disaster response to interview did not have an apparent impact on participants' ability to recall details. Recollections were clear and meticulous, regardless of when the disaster occurred. One participant's words were especially heart rendering but insightful as he shared the following comments about his memories:

> I remember … that memory is almost like HD [high definition] … crystal clear … I remember the time of day, the temperature, how fast the breeze was blowing … people running back and forth … I can see their faces sometimes … when they are coming down the hill … and the looks on their faces … and how they are looking for some hope or understanding.

It is significant not only for who the participants were or the contents of the themes to follow but also the way in which their stories were shared. All began with a discussion of military culture, their lens in the world that so clearly defined them. In their telling of disaster experiences, they compared those lived events with their knowledge of war and combat and military life and training.

THEMES AND EXEMPLARS

Six themes emerged and were identifiable across all the transcripts. These themes were nature of war versus nature of disaster, known versus unknown, structured

Table 1
Participant demographic characteristics (n = 23)

Characteristics	n	%
Sex		
Male	10	(43.4)
Female	13	(56.5)
Branch of service		
Air Force	11	(47.8)
Army	8	(34.7)
Navy	2	(8.7)
US Public Health Service	2	(8.7)
Nature of disasters		
Natural	22	(95.6)
Man-made	5	(21.7)
Number of disaster responses		
1	21	(91.3)
2	5	(21.7)
3	1	(4.3)

Table 2	
Overview of disasters discussed and year of occurrence	
Disaster	**Year**
Loma Prieta earthquake	1989
Red River Valley flood	1997
Adana, Ceyhan earthquake	1998
Hurricane Mitch	1998
US Embassy bombing, Nairobi	1998
Pentagon attack	2001
Washington DC anthrax attacks	2001
Hurricane Ivan	2004
Bethel, Alaska flu epidemic	2004
Soto Cano Air Base crash	2005
Hurricane Katrina	2005
Hurricane Rita	2005
Muzaffarabad, Pakistan earthquake	2005
St Louis, MO tornado	2006
Hurricane Gustav	2008
Hurricane Ike	2008
Tropical Storm Hannah	2008

versus chaos, prepared versus making do, being strong versus expressing emotion, and existential growth.

Nature of War Versus Nature of Disaster

The participants shared their description of the differences between war and disaster and what combat itself actually represented. One nurse elaborated in her opening remarks:

> There's a difference in expectations during wartime. I had been to war…We knew what should be done and what our mission was…[but] no matter how much you think you are prepared for Mother Nature to come in and knock you on your butt, you have no idea what you are dealing with.

Another nurse stated the differences he recognized:

> When we were over there [war] it's organized, you know exactly what [patients] you are getting…where you are moving them to…but over here [disaster] information is limited, disorganized, you didn't know where you were going until you were rolling.

Known Versus Unknown

Participants expressed what they knew about war and how to fight a war, which was substantial. But when compared with a disaster, they articulated they were greatly unprepared to confront this entity. They shared that there was a scarcity of information and lack of preparation before the response.

> [In war] you know exactly what your job is … [but in disaster] there is a level of uncertainty … you don't know where people are… we didn't know what we were going to get when we got there…you didn't know.

[In war, we were given the training, so we knew what to expect ... they told us ... [what conditions were like] before we got there ...what to expect ... but in disasters, we knew very little before we got there.

Structured Versus Chaos

In the military, there are policies and procedures that are preplanned and followed; but during disaster response, all that structure is absent initially.

[In the disaster] it was just like chaos. You are so used to structure and suddenly there is none ... everything that you knew doesn't exist anymore ... that piece of the puzzle that's normally organized before you get there doesn't exist anymore.

When "[We were preparing for war] we had people, we had stuff, we had training ... [but] it was very chaotic and ever changing in a disaster."

Prepared Versus Making Do

The nurses indicated that war is something they train for and are prepared for when they receive the orders to deploy; but on entering the disaster areas, the nurses spoke of having to be innovative and doing the best they could when aiding the victims.

[In the disaster] ... we used plastic covers [from our packing supplies] to make isolation rooms ... for traction devices ... we used filled 5-gallon water jugs and bottles of [povidone-iodine] Betadine.

You know, you would try to help them but it was ... a very bare bones operation.

You are overwhelmed with not having all the supplies you need and ... you just do the best you can with what you have.

Being Strong Versus Expressing Emotion

Military members are expected to demonstrate strength and perseverance in all aspects of their duty. Emotional endurance is included in that mindset. However, within the world of disaster, the participants openly expressed their emotions.

[Those of us who serve in the military] we are supposed to be the strong ones ... but at the end ... it becomes a bit more difficult [to keep it inside, it builds up] because you [just] can't share everything that goes on there [in the disaster].

If it [disaster] doesn't touch you, something of that magnitude, then you've probably got some other problems.

There was tremendous benefit [from] verbalizing your feelings ... that is how we dealt with it ... came together ... With locked arms ... we would spend time just talking about our feelings and our memories.

Existential Growth

As the participants reexamined their thoughts regarding their experience and the outcomes of the disaster, they realized they had grown as a result of their efforts; they had reached a higher level of awareness. They gained an insight into the bigger picture of life; they stepped out of themselves and viewed the events and the outcomes of the disaster through a new lens of being in the world.

It kind of reshaped my thinking about catastrophic events...until you see the big picture, you don't appreciate it...it is a very enlightening experience...it is a very gut-wrenching experience in appreciation...appreciation of how people's lives can just be simply, totally...disrupted...sometimes we think we have experienced everything, but by the grace of God go I.

I came away with a lot more ... awareness of what goes on out there ... what I experienced 3 years ago continues to stay with me ... to improve how I ... look at other people and not to be judgmental ... to take people for who they are and understand the situation where they are coming from.

DISCUSSION

The military nurses' experiences of disaster response were concentrated in the phenomenological world of others. The contextual ground of the military culture was a focal point against which they attempted to orient themselves within the disaster experiences. However, they quickly realized that this was not always possible because war/combat and disaster response were two very different experiences. Drawing on previous combat training and knowledge gained from wartime deployments, the participants described the diversities of serving within the disaster environment. Yet, regardless of the disaster event, military branch, or individual rank of the participants, it was clear there were numerous similarities that came to light in their stories. Time from disaster response to participation in the study did not deter the nurses from providing a rich description regarding their experiences of responding to and sometimes being in a disaster that will be forever ingrained in their memories. These memories led to lessons learned that warrants addressing.

BEHAVIORAL HEALTH LESSONS LEARNED

Emotional impact was significant and undervalued. The stress from the response actions far exceeded what was expected. Their experiences were so overwhelming that being strong did not work. The participants stated that individuals who had not been involved in their disaster experiences could not possibly understand what they had endured. To cope, they became their own stress teams, discussing their anxieties and things they had witnessed throughout the disaster deployment. These stress teams continue even into present day as some of the participants remain in contact with each other. The nurses mentioned that living conditions were worse than in previous combat deployments. They shared that violence was expected during war but never anticipated in disaster response. They were not prepared for this type of danger. The reduced organization and typical efficiency familiar in combat was absent and caused even greater concerns.

Military nurses are at risk for experiencing emotional distress and could potentially demonstrate signs of compassion fatigue and behavioral health issues. Many of the nurses specifically mentioned the lack of adequate debriefing and ongoing emotional support on their return. Therefore, reintegration into their regular duties and typical roles was a factor. Behavioral health concerns for responders are noted in the literature and indicate responders are at risk following traumatic issues, which supports the outcomes of this study. During Hurricane Celia, stress, physical demands, safety, and lack of supplies were issues identified from the nurses who were interviewed. They shared that watching the suffering of the victims and enduring the chaos was difficult.[15] One nurse expressed the human devastation he witnessed, how "just every 3 minutes, someone died." Another nurse remarked how she worked around the clock for several days trying to sand bag and protect their military field site before and following the hurricane. Several nurses told how there were so many people just being "herded through the shelters" for evacuation, there was very little space between the individuals.

Dickerson and colleagues[16] interviewed nurses regarding their experiences of responding to the attack on the world traded center. Traumatic stress emerged as a theme when nurses recalled witnessing firefighters recovering body parts from the rubble, the grief and mourning of disaster workers, and the smell of death. Boivin[17] shared a summary of 2 personal interviews conducted with the chief nurse of the Pentagon health clinic, narratives in which the nurse described her perspective of the events of September 11. Like the civilian nurses in the Dickerson and colleagues[16] research, the chief nurse reported emotional pain at the realization of a disaster's enormous power to claim lives and lingering feelings of sadness. Adams[18] emphasizes the vulnerability of both volunteer and paid responders following a disaster event. She notes that the respondent should be aware of his or her own needs, particularly emotional distress. Similarly, Whall and colleagues[19] stress the importance of psychological factors in well-being.

As one nurse in this recent study indicated:

Poof, we are back ... transported back ... expected to go on with our life ... to go on with life [when] ... no one else has experienced that you have experienced...how do we all really deal [with it].

Thus, the military services need to advance policy supporting behavioral health in disaster response for the military personnel. Behavioral health support has been established for the victims of disasters. Combat stress teams are embedded in combat units; but unfortunately, these types of teams were not available during the nurses' disaster responses. Another issue that caused increased stress was that they were going into the known. They had no idea what they would find once they arrived; there was no indication of what logistical support they would have, if any, or even what their roles would be fulfilling once they were in the area. Several of these nurses served roles not typically expected. From filling sandbags and completing forms to help link loved ones with the deceased and building huts, all of these unknowns tasked their mental reservoirs. Another issue that led to their emotional stress was the lack of communication before and during the response efforts.

COMMUNICATION LESSONS LEARNED

During any disastrous event, crisis communication becomes a key component to relay essential information to the individuals within the disaster area. Unfortunately, communication disruptions and failures are an inescapable component of crisis, most often attributable to the chaos that ensues following the precipitating event.[20] The medical response to the attack on the Pentagon was examined and noted the lack of emergency communication capability between the numerous treatment facilities.[21]

Similarly, the participants of this current study expressed a lack of communication that led to disorganization and hindered disaster response efforts. One of the nurses pointed out her "fear of being left behind" as she was trying to locate and join a unit she did not know. Nurses spoke of how inadequate/flawed communication led to supply shortages due to wrong items being shipped, which snowballed into increased disorganization. One nurse explained how she was deployed into the disaster area without her command having any information about who she needed to contact on arrival. Another nurse stated his team had no idea what to expect with regard to the disaster, as no communication was coming out of the city before their deployment.

Inaccurate information transmitted to the public sapped morale of the responders. The media, at times, impeded the response actions and provisions of safe care as they toured the disaster sites. The participants described how media reporting caused mental anguish among the disaster responders. They emphasized how the negative reports discredited the positive things that were being done. Several mentioned they (the nurses) were working as hard and quickly as they could but were reported as being slow and uncaring. One nurse mentioned how a media broadcaster would cause the crowd to become unruly with his news broadcast. A third nurse spoke of how she refrained from watching the news, as she was engulfed in the disaster and hearing the biased news reports increased her stress and anxiety. Collaborative efforts between the media and responders are needed and produce a stronger front, thus, decreasing fear, frustration, and anxiety.[20,22] Therefore, the findings of this present study agree with that of the previous literature.

Media need limits when entering disaster zones. Nurses need training in working with the media to garner the significance of setting effective limits or boundaries while rendering care during these chaotic times. Currently, civilian reporters are imbedded with combat teams to cover happenings during wars. Consequently, those individuals have a better understanding of the efforts that are provided. Perhaps it is feasible to have civilian journalists accompany military units as they move to provide a disaster response. Several other areas regarding lessons learned surfaced during the interviews. These areas included education, practice, and training.

EDUCATION LESSONS LEARNED

Two articles indicated the necessity for disaster education to be added to nursing curriculum.[23,24] Even though the need has been recognized in the literature, very few colleges and universities have incorporated disaster awareness and disaster response courses into the curriculum. Findings of this study continue to support the addition of disaster response courses to nursing curricula as identified by scholarly works. Several participants mentioned problems with coordination in disasters. The Federal Emergency Management Agency's courses regarding incident command and working with nongovernmental agencies would be beneficial. Military units have begun conducting disaster drills with civilian partners. One of the nurses mentioned concerns of hazardous materials noted in the disaster area. Hazardous material courses would also be beneficial.

Military nurses need disaster-specific training. It became quite obvious that combat readiness was not equal to disaster readiness. Adding disaster education to basic nursing education at all levels would serve as an excellent foundation. Even more, there is a need for military leaders with advanced degrees in disaster management that would indeed be invaluable. Mandated military courses should consider adding a disaster response element into their lesson plans.

PRACTICE AND TRAINING LESSONS LEARNED

Military nurses often practice mass casualties each year based on a disaster scenario; however, this may or may not include civilian-military partnerships that is imperative for disaster response. Often, the scenarios practiced are within the main hospital or have the main hospital support during the exercise. As indicated by the nurses in this study, sophisticated, even basic materials or equipment may be absent.

We used a version of jet fuel to heat water … cooks used it … the OR [operation room] used it … our equipment was serialized with fire.

Therefore, much of the training must include the use of primitive equipment, basic hands-on skills and, potentially, altered standards of care as supplies dwindle. As there is a difference between cultures and traditions within US borders, this is even more so in foreign countries. Understanding culture and traditions in any disaster area is an essential element to ensure a successful, collaborative response effort.

SUMMARY

Disasters, whether natural or man-made, persist worldwide and will do so into the future. Although not the initial responders, military personnel continually assist with these traumatic events. Among these military personnel will be nurses who share responsibilities in the response efforts. This study examined military nurses' experiences of disaster response. Their narratives included both positive and negative aspects of what their journeys entailed. As they moved into the disaster zone, they became a cohesive unit, leaning on one another through the hardships and the good times. Those bonds created still exist today. Many nurses indicated that this was the first time they had spoken of their experiences outside of their deployment groups. Their response efforts provided a unique opportunity to learn something about themselves and the people around them. Moreover, the knowledge gained from this study adds to the body of disaster nursing literature and that of military studies. Through their stories, we recognize that there are similarities between combat and disaster deployments. However, we now know there are also many compelling differences. More importantly, this study provided lessons learned that have the potential to assist in preparing for the next disaster response.

REFERENCES

1. Kreps GA. Disasters as systemic event and social catalyst. Int J Mass Emerg Disasters 1995;13:255–84.
2. Abbott EB, Hetzel OJ. A legal guide to homeland security and emergency management for state and local governments. Chicago: American Bar Association; 2005.
3. Komnenich P, Feller C. Disaster nursing. Annu Rev Nurs Res 1991;9:123–34.
4. International Committee of the Red Cross. From the battle of Solferino to the eve of the First World War. 2004. Available at: http://www.icrc.org/eng/resources/documents/misc/57jnvp.htm. Accessed March 28, 2016.
5. Sarnecky MT. A history of the army nurse corps. Philadelphia: University of Pennsylvania Press; 1999.
6. West IJ, Clark C. The army nurse corps and operation restore hope. Mil Med 1995;160:179–83.
7. Wong W, Brandt L, Keenan ME. Massachusetts general hospital in operation unified assistance for tsunami relief in Banda Ache Indonesia. Mil Med 2006;171:S37–9.
8. Elleman BA. Waves of hope: Navy's response to the tsunami in northern Indonesia. 2008. 2007. Available at: http://www.dtic.mil/cgi-bin/GetTRDoc?AD=ADA463367&Location=U2&doc=GetTRDoc.pdf. Accessed March 28, 2016.

9. Pakistan earthquake: A review of the civil-military dimensions of the international response. 2005. Available at: https://wss.apan.org/432/Files/Resources/References/Lessons%20Learned/Pakistan%20Earthquake.doc. Accessed March 28, 2016.

10. Auerbach PS, Noris RL, Menon AS, et al. Civil-military collaboration in the initial medical response to the earthquake in Haiti. N Engl J Med 2010;10:e31–4.

11. Keck Z. U. S. Military vs. Hurricane Sandy: with the eastern U.S. under siege thanks to Hurricane Sandy the U.S. military has turned its disaster response capabilities inward. 2012. Available at: http://thediplomat.com/2012/10/u-s-military-vs-hurricane-sandy/. Accessed March 28, 2016.

12. Jacoby CH, Grass FL. Dual-status, single purpose: a unified response to hurricane sandy. 2013. Available at: http://www.ang.af.mil/news/story.asp?id=123339975. Accessed March 28, 2016.

13. Almonte AL. Humanitarian nursing challenges: a grounded theory study. Mil Med 2009;174:479–85.

14. Thomas S, Pollio H. Listening to patients: a phenomenological approach to nursing research and practice. New York: Springer; 2002.

15. Laube J. Psychological reactions of nurses in disaster. Nurs Res 1973;22:343–7.

16. Dickerson SS, Jezewski M, Nelson-Tuttle C, et al. Nursing at ground zero: experiences during and after September 11 World Trade Cent attack. J N Y State Nurses Assoc 2002;33:27–33.

17. Boivin J. Pentagon nurse quells chaos of terrorist. Nurs Spectr (Wash D C) 2001;11:19–36.

18. Adams L. Mental health needs of disaster volunteers: a plea for awareness. Perspect Psychiatr Care 2007;43:52–4.

19. Whall AL, YunHee S, Colling KB. A nightingale-based model for dementia care and its relevance for Korean nursing. Nurs Sci Q 1999;12:319–23.

20. Sonnier S. Communication in a disaster. In: Adelman DS, Legg TJ, editors. Disaster nursing: a handbook for practice. Subury (MA): Jones and Bartlett; 2009. p. 133–4.

21. Wang D, Sava J, Sample G, et al. The pentagon and 9/11. Crit Care Med 2005;33:S42–7.

22. Nacos B. Crisis communication: the role of the media. In: Veenema TG, editor. Disaster nursing and emergency preparedness: for chemical, biological and radiological terrorism and other hazards. New York: Springer; 2007. p. 119–34.

23. Neal MV. Disaster nursing preparation. Report of a pilot project conducted in four schools of nursing and one hospital nursing service. New York: National League for Nursing; 1963 (ERIC Document Reproduction Service No. ED026477).

24. Littleton-Kearney MT, Slepski LA. Directions for disaster nursing education in the United States. Crit Care Nurs Clin North Am 2008;20:103–9.

Wildfire Disasters and Nursing

Patricia Frohock Hanes, PhD, MSN, MAEd, MS-DPEM, RN, CNE

KEYWORDS

- Nursing education • Disaster nursing • Disasters • Emergency preparedness
- Wildfires

KEY POINTS

- Nurses must take an active role in preparing personally and professionally for wildfires and other disasters.
- Major nursing organizations support disaster preparedness and education.
- Disaster education should be an integral part of nursing programs at all levels.
- Health effects from wildfires can progress to long-term health issues, both physical and psychological.

WILDFIRE DISASTERS AND NURSING

Wildfires in California are increasing and concomitant health effects, which, although recognized by many investigators, have not been examined in the context of nursing.[1–8] Because most nurses live in the region in which they are employed, wildfires have an impact on nurses personally and professionally. It is essential for nurses to understand the implications for health care related to this disaster; the impact extends beyond first responders and public health nurses to those in nearly all areas of nursing. First, however, nurses must understand the larger context surrounding wildfires: the disaster cycle (mitigation, preparedness, response, and recovery) and nursing's roles in each part of that cycle, the position of major nursing organizations on disasters and nursing, and human and environmental factors that contribute to the increasing frequency and severity of wildfires. Nursing's roles in disasters and wildfires have not been explored in much depth outside of caring for those with traumatic injuries. There is much that nurses can and should do in all phases of disaster; this exploratory article provides an overview of factors contributing to wildfires, health effects, and the roles of nurses in wildfire disasters.

Financial Disclosures: None.
Azusa Pacific University School of Nursing, 701 East Foothill Boulevard, Azusa, CA 91702, USA
E-mail address: phanes@apu.edu

PRECURSORS TO DISASTER

To truly understand the events leading up to the disastrous wildfires in California, it is important to recognize 4 contributing phenomena: drought, winds, climate change, and spreading urbanization (each with its own unique health effects). In recent years, California has suffered from a historic multiyear drought. Wells and reservoirs have run dry. Lack of planning, extensive development, and other factors have led to so much water use that the land is sinking up to a foot (30 cm) a year due to depletion of the water table.[9] Farmers who grow crops that supply the entire United States have watched their water allotments shrink. Larger cities have implemented strict water rationing; those with private water systems are forced to import water. Entire towns have been closed due to lack of drinking water, disrupting lives, separating families, and impacting health. There are economic disasters as well; home values plummet and businesses go bankrupt. People cannot afford adequate health insurance. Drought causes a cascade of events leading to extended fire "seasons" and catastrophic fires. According to the State of California Drought Web site, the entire state is currently in an "extreme drought" condition that one rainy season cannot rectify.[6,10]

Santa Ana winds (called by other names in different areas: chinooks in the Rocky Mountains and foehns in other regions) are dry, hot winds that blow from east to west over the mountains surrounding Southern California. As air comes over the mountains it dries out and compresses, rushing down mountainsides and heating. Winds range from 25 mph to greater than 60 mph, with gusts even higher.[6–11] These gale-force winds are strong enough to blow over full-grown oak trees, cinder block walls, and fences. The low, single-digit humidity dries vegetation quickly, in particular grasses and other small vegetation, and desiccates soil, leading to increased fuel for fast-moving fires. People with respiratory diseases, in particular asthma, are affected by increased dust particles in the air[12] and radio warnings are issued to keep vulnerable persons indoors.

Climate change, caused by increasing greenhouse gases, is leading to higher temperatures and less rainfall in California. According to the National Resources Defense Council[13] and the California Department of Water Resources,[14] multiple health effects are related to climate change, including those related to lack of water due to drought, heat-related illnesses, infectious disease, and health effects from air pollution and extreme weather, including an increase in wildfires.

Southern California alone has a population of more than 22 million people and includes the major metropolitan areas of Los Angeles and San Diego and densely populated surrounding communities with varied demographics.[15] Areas near mountains and Southern California's 4 national forests are highly desirable places to live. As populations increase, communities are encroaching into wildland areas for either status or affordability. This expanding wildland-urban interface (WUI) leads to increasing damage from wildfires due to wind-driven fires blowing down canyons to areas with limited defensibility and restricted accessibility due to either topography or lack of major roads. Living in WUI areas can place people at risk for dangers from wildfires, either directly from smoke and flames or later from dangers of flooding and mudslides after heavy seasonal rains rush down denuded hillsides (**Figs. 1–4**).[15]

DISASTER IN THE MAKING

It was January 16, 2014, and an unusually warm day in the Los Angeles area with temperatures approximately 82°F (27°C). There were severe drought conditions due to a historic lack of rainfall for 2 years. That day, dry offshore Santa Ana winds were predicted. Residents, particularly in the mountains and foothills, are always on alert

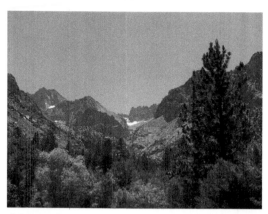

Fig. 1. Inyo National Forest. The topography makes some areas of California almost impossible to access on foot during fires. The population is sparse, resulting in less human damage during wildfires. Note heavy brush and trees. (*Courtesy of* Dr Patricia Hanes.)

when there are Santa Anas because wind gusts can reach hurricane force. Any spark can become a firestorm in minutes with the combination of high winds and extremely dry vegetation. Often fires are started by humans, accidentally, carelessly, or purposely. A fire was started that day by an illegal campfire that went out of control in the steep mountains above Azusa and Glendora, 2 Los Angeles suburbs with large WUI communities.

Just a short distance away were Azusa Pacific University and Citrus College, with a total combined student population of more than 23,000 students.[16,17] At housing developments more than 7 miles (11 km) from the university and approximately 9 miles (14.5 km) from the fire, the air was stifling and smoky. Small ash particles dusted any horizontal surface. Schools near the fire were closing, either due to their proximity to the fire or so they could be used as evacuation centers. Citrus College, a community

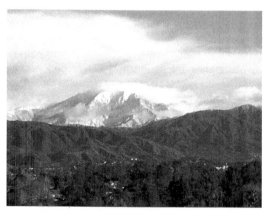

Fig. 2. View of San Gabriel Mountains demonstrating WUI. Houses continue to be built into canyons in heavily populated suburbs of Los Angeles. This picture was taken approximately 8 miles (12.8 km) from the base of the foothills. Note clouds coming over mountain demonstrating wind effect. Steep canyons increase wind speed and force during a Santa Ana wind event, increasing the rapid spread and severity of fires. (*Courtesy of* Dr Patricia Hanes.)

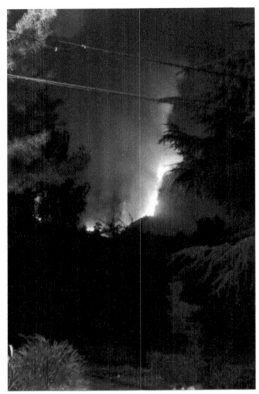

Fig. 3. The San Gabriel Mountains from a friend's backyard during the Altadena fire in 2009. (*Courtesy of* Dr Marsha Fowler.)

college whose students are all commuters, closed to keep the roads clear. Although flames could be seen at the far end of the road that lead to the mountains in front of Azusa Pacific University, the difficult decision was made to keep the campus open. With approximately 3500 residential students, many without cars, evacuations—unless absolutely necessary—could put students in danger and tax the already overburdened local road and traffic systems. Students and some staff remained on campus but there were significant health and safety concerns, especially for the nurses in the university health center, as the sky became darker, smokier, and more ash-filled and as the fire raged closer and closer to the more heavily populated and industrial areas on the valley floor.

The closest local hospital, Foothill Presbyterian Hospital, activated its emergency operations center. If there were major injuries or medical emergencies, this would be the place where patients would likely be transported. There were other worries, however. If the fire crossed major roads as it roared down the mountain, the hospital itself might be in jeopardy. Although this was unlikely, preliminary preparations were made to evacuate the hospital quickly should the need arise. News outlets were clamoring for information on this as well as the main story about the fires; nurses entering the hospital were asked to comment.

The fire raged for days, causing massive evacuations, burning homes, and fouling the air. This led to exacerbations of chronic illnesses and flare-ups of respiratory diseases, such as asthma. Although the areas immediately adjacent to the fire were

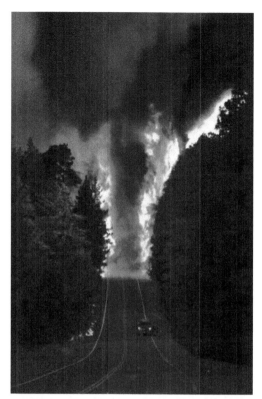

Fig. 4. Old Fire on mountain road east of Los Angeles, 2003. (*From* CAL FIRE. California Fire Siege of 2003: The story. Available at: http://www.fire.ca.gov/downloads/2003 FireStory Internet.pdf. Accessed June 29, 2016.)

evacuated, others were still open, even though the air was filled with smoke and ash and flames were clearly visible from miles away.[18]

This scenario is repeated every year in California as the dry, desert climate and Santa Ana winds converge to place the area at high risk during fire season, which often begins after the winter rains (if there are any) end and the area begins to dry out. The season can extend into December or later. There is no set date, but declaring fire season open enables assets to be acquired and staged (**Box 1**, **Fig. 5**).

UNDERSTANDING WILDFIRE DISASTERS

A wildfire is defined as "a brush or wildland fire burning out of control over great geographic range" and is considered a meteorologic event because it arises "closely associated with weather conditions," such as low humidity, high winds, dry lightning, and unstable air.[3] Wildfire disasters can be caused by nature or by human action. The scale of wildfires can be very large or relatively small, of short duration or long. Wildfires can be associated with secondary disasters, such as the mass casualty incident that occurred when a fast-moving wildfire overtook cars and trucks on a busy Southern California freeway in 2015. Secondary disasters can be delayed, as with flash flooding down fire-denuded hillsides, risking lives and property. Primary disasters, such as earthquakes, can cause other, secondary disasters, such as wildfires that strip hillsides, leading to later flooding and mudslides. Disasters become complex

---

Box 1
Resources, reports, and videos

- News video of fire: "Firefight Continues in 1700 acre Colby Fire; Blaze 30% Contained" at http://ktla.com/2014/01/16/firefighters-battling-brushfire-north-of-glendora/.

- Online article on mass casualty event due to wildfire burning cars on Southern California freeway: https://www.rt.com/usa/310144-500-acre-california-brush-fire/; Accessed June 29, 2016.

- News reports on Fort McMurray fire: http://www.bbc.com/news/world-us-canada-36199993; Accessed May 4, 2016.

- An example of a Web site for wildfire risk forecasting from the California Wildland Fire Coordinating Group: http://www.preventwildfireca.org/Wildfire-Forecasting/

- Wildfire teaching tool from Ready.Gov: www.fema.gov/media-library-data/79a16f6b198fa8 7ba7b0255838c54904/FEMA_FS_wildfire_508.pdf; Accessed June 27, 2016.

- Active fire maps in the US and Canada provided by the US Department of Agriculture Forest Service: http://activefiremaps.fs.fed.us/.

- Video from the California EPA Air Resources Board on "Protecting Yourself from Wildfire Smoke" to learn about educating people on potential health effects from wildfire smoke: http://www.arb.ca.gov/videos/impacts_of_smoke.htm.

- Examples of information on recovery and protecting health by the California EPA; see CalEPA fire response: http://www.calepa.ca.gov/Disaster/Fire/.

---

humanitarian events when the initial wildfire disaster leads to other disasters, such as burning of entire towns causing mass evacuations as seen in the Canadian 2011 Slave Lake and 2016 Fort McMurray fires. These massive fires can lead to loss of local infrastructure and lack of essential services, such as water, sanitation, and health care. This is an even larger problem in rural areas, where additional supports can be very far away (see **Box 1**).[2,19]

Although specific wildfires are unpredictable, communities can assess their risk for wildfires using readily available tools to mitigate against and prepare for wildfires. For example, one hospital in San Diego County, California, assessed wildfires as a major threat. Going beyond the usual plan for increasing capacity, they trained for full hospital evacuation. In the wildfires of 2007, fast-moving wildfires threatened the area and the hospital and nearby skilled nursing facility were evacuated (see **Box 1**).[1]

Wildfire Assistance

Disasters begin locally but the response increases as the event enlarges. Many localities have mutual aid agreements with other communities. As areas are overwhelmed, regional and/or state assistance may be requested. States in some regions form compacts to render mutual aid. Assets, such as water-dropping aircraft, fire engines, or medical supplies, may be contracted for or requested as part of a memorandum of understanding and deployed as needed. Volunteer organizations, such as the ARC, Salvation Army, and several early-responding nongovernmental organizations, respond with resources, such as shelters (some with basic medical care), basic necessities (eg, food, blankets, and toiletries), and communications to assist survivors with reunification. Many private companies have response plans where they help communities by providing needed supplies. For example, some beer bottling plants have plans to convert to bottled water to supply local communities should the need arise. Other companies, such as big-box stores, may provide goods and services.

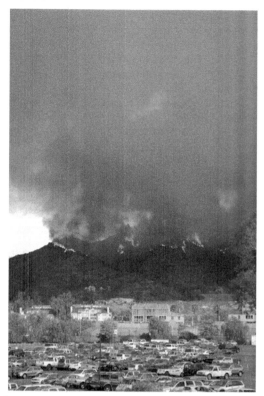

Fig. 5. The Colby fire, January, 2014, from Azusa Pacific University in Azusa, California. (*From* Yu AZ. Colby Fire burns near campus. January 16, 2014. Available at: http://www.theclause.org/2014/01/colby-fire-burns-near-campus/. Accessed April 4, 2016. Photo credit: Kimberly Smith.)

In the disastrous 2003 Southern California fire season, 750,043 acres were burned, 3710 homes were lost, and 24 people died between October 21 and November 4. Firefighters and citizens were exposed to flames, smoke, high temperatures, heavy winds, and falling debris. Heavy traffic, damaged power lines, steep terrain, and burning structures posed additional hazards. A state psychiatric hospital was evacuated. One hospital in a mountain community was evacuated, along with the rest of the town. Crews, working 48 hours without relief, were exhausted. With all fire assets deployed to the wildfires, one city had no one left at any fire station to answer routine calls. Communities were left without power and some had no access to water. These fires were rated at Preparedness Level 5, the highest level, where the fire danger is extreme and national assets are mobilized.[20] As multiple fires raged out of control and resources were overwhelmed, additional state, national, and military assets were deployed. National Guard helicopters were requested from neighboring states. Fire engines came from local, state, and national sources; volunteers responded.

Phases of Disaster and Levels of Prevention

Most nurses are familiar with levels of prevention: primary, secondary, and tertiary. Primary prevention represents health-promoting, illness-preventing activities. Secondary prevention is early detection, such as assessing wildfire vulnerability, whereas tertiary prevention is controlling and limiting complications and casualties.[21] These levels align somewhat with the stages of disaster and disaster nursing competencies.[22] The Federal Emergency Management Agency and other agencies have used different names for the phases of disaster but commonly used terms are mitigation, preparedness, response, and recovery (**Fig. 6**).[23] The goal of understanding the disaster phases is to decrease effects of wildfires and increase community resilience. This is not an activity for just one organization or individual; to be effective, it must involve the whole community working together. Nurses need to analyze their responsibilities in different phases of wildfire disasters (**Table 1**). They have roles in preparing for and responding to wildfires and can help increase community resilience through participating in mitigation and recovery activities.

Mitigation

Mitigation activities of particular interest to nurses involve health promotion activities, professional and public education regarding health effects due to wildfires, and preparing for public health needs, for example, by developing additional health care sites to divert subacute patients from overwhelmed acute care facilities.[24] Hospital disaster plans must reflect risk from wildfires and include plans for evacuation. Nurses must analyze the practicality and effectiveness of those plans and be ready to implement them should the need arise (see **Box 1**; **Figs. 7** and **8**).

Preparedness

Preparedness refers to activities contributing to readiness to respond and recover; it needs to occur both personally and professionally. Nurses who are not prepared personally have difficulty responding to a disaster. Professionally, preparedness also includes developing community and workplace wildfire policies and procedures, and training, evaluating, and modifying activities in accordance with governmental and industry standards.[24] There is a need for volunteer nurses to engage in professional preparedness activities by registering with volunteer organizations like the Medical Reserve Corp or the American Red Cross (ARC); in wildfire disasters, nurses are needed, for example, in shelters and aid stations. Understanding potential health

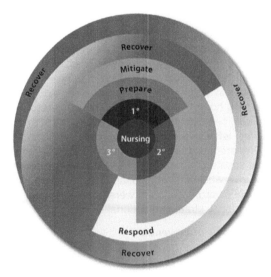

Fig. 6. The disaster cycle related to primary, secondary, and tertiary levels of care and nursing. (*Courtesy of* Dr Patricia Hanes and David McGill.)

Table 1			
The disaster management cycle, wildfires, and nursing			
	Goal	Examples	Sample Questions Related to Wildfires and Nursing
Mitigation Level of care: primary, secondary	Minimize effects of disaster	Hazard vulnerability Analysis, public education	How vulnerable is my location/organization to fire and its after-effects? Are we in a fire zone? Do we have a functional, detailed evacuation plan? How can I prepare for clients' health needs in the event of a fire? Do they have the knowledge to prepare an evacuation kit with adequate medications, oxygen, etc.? What health-related resources are available to my facility/community to prepare for a large wildfire event? Do we have mutual aid agreements with other facilities/communities?
Preparedness Level of care: primary	Planning how to respond	Preparedness plans, gathering and storing supplies, education, exercises and training	Do I have a personal plan for fire evacuation? Does my facility have enough supplies if employees and clients need sheltering? How can we access more supplies if needed? Would some of my clients have difficulty evacuating in case of a fire?
Response Level of care: secondary, tertiary	Lessen hazards and loss from a disaster	First aid, search and rescue, emergency relief	Is my facility prepared for a mass casualty event? How would we treat severe burns? How prepared are we to care for clients' and employees' health needs during the fire event (eg, poor air quality, staffing needs, etc.)? When do we decide to evacuate? Is our evacuation plan feasible? Could we evacuate the entire facility if necessary? How? Where?

(continued on next page)

Table 1
(continued)

	Goal	Examples	Sample Questions Related to Wildfires and Nursing

Recovery
Level of care:
  secondary,
  tertiary,
  primary
	Returning community to "normal"	Temporary housing, loans and grants, long-term medical care	How can I help my community recover?
			Is my community prepared to address the long-term health effects related to a fire disaster?
			Do we have sufficient resources to address psychological recovery?

Adapted from Warfield C. The disaster management cycle. Available at: http://www.gdrc.org/uem/disasters/1-dm_cycle.html. Accessed March 16, 2016.

effects from wildfires enables nurses to help their families, clients, and communities to understand what they need to do to protect their health and to be safe during a wildfire. For example, people, whether evacuating or not, need to be prepared for poor air quality, sometimes far from the actual fire zone. Nurses, in addition to educating clients, can help develop special accommodations that may be needed for people affected by poor air quality (see **Box 1**; **Fig. 9**).

Response
Nurses' responses to disasters depend on many factors: the type of response needed, their professional roles, whether it is a local disaster or if they are coming with an aid organization, and their own personal preparation and obligations (see **Table 1**). Nurses must understand the context of wildfires to better care for civilians and responders. In the 2003 Southern California wildfires, nurses prepared to rapidly evacuate a large general hospital and a smaller children's hospital.[5] In 2007, nurses were part of a team that successfully evacuated a hospital and skilled nursing facility.[1] Rural nurses in Australia traveled to patients' homes after a massive 2009 bushfire (wildfire) and found rubble where patients' homes had been[25] while hospital nurses, attempting

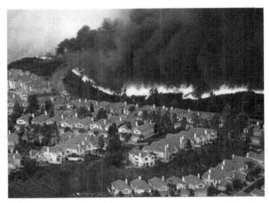

Fig. 7. Building in WUI areas causes risk to people and property. Health effects can continue long after fire has been extinguished. (*From* CAL FIRE-FEMA. Available at: http://osfm.fire.ca.gov/codedevelopment/wildfireprotectionbuildingconstruction. Accessed June 27, 2016.)

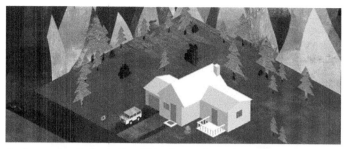

Fig. 8. Protecting property from fire. This picture from the Lassen County (CA) Fire Safe Council shows brush clearance around the home. (*From* Lassen County Fire Safe Council. Available at: http://www.lassenfiresafecouncil.org/. Accessed June 27, 2016.)

to discharge patients, had to find shelter for patients whose homes had burned.[26] At this writing, the ARC is asking for nurses to deploy to a large wildfire in Central California (see **Box 1**; **Figs. 10** and **11**).

Recovery

Finally, recovery aims at helping communities return to functional levels as quickly as possible (resilience). This often involves adjusting to a new normal, particularly when there has been mass destruction, as in the aforementioned Slave Lake and Fort McMurray fires, and also when losses are on a smaller scale, particularly when there have been deaths. This is the longest phase and can last a decade or more. Recovery is facilitated when communities work together to be prepared[24] (see **Table 1**). Part of recovery is supporting caregivers, as when Australian nurses discussed the toll the bushfires had taken on them emotionally and physically. Often, especially in smaller communities, patients are neighbors and sometimes family. In 2003, when a San Diego nurse was evacuating, her car was overtaken by fire; her daughter died but she and her other child survived.[5] An Australian psychiatric nurse who was a victim in the 2009 bushfires emphasized the importance of early mental health interventions (see **Box 1**; **Figs. 12** and **13**).[27]

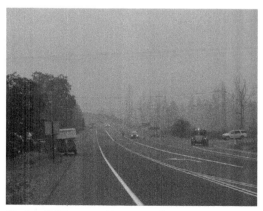

Fig. 9. Poor air quality in wildfire zone. (*Courtesy of* Larry Masterman, EMT-P, Medford, Oregon, Director of Emergency Services.)

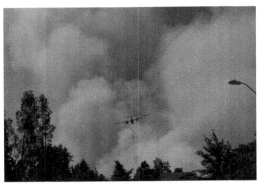

Fig. 10. Responders place themselves at risk when flying into hazardous, smoky conditions. (*Courtesy of* Larry Masterman, EMT-P, Medford, Oregon, Director of Emergency Services.)

WILDFIRES IN CALIFORNIA

When fueled by gusting winds, embers can be blown for miles, landing in trees, on roofs, and under the eaves of homes, burning neighborhoods seemingly out of reach of the ignition point. Although wildfires themselves cause great damage and injury, secondary disasters can also occur after the fires, for example, mudslides, flooding, and diseases, such as coccidioidomycosis, a fungus endemic to the dry regions of California (**Fig. 14, Table 2; Table 4**). More than 80% of wildfires are caused by people.[8] Records from the California Department of Forestry and Fire Protection (CAL FIRE) from 1923 to 2013 show that humans directly caused at least 50% of the 20 deadliest and costliest fires in California and at least 40% of the largest fires (some fires were under investigation or causes were unknown). Other major causes included lightning and arcing power lines (see **Fig. 14**).[28]

TYPES OF WILDFIRES

Recent research in wildfires has uncovered 2 distinct types of wildfires in California: those spread by Santa Ana winds and those occurring in the dry, hot summer season.

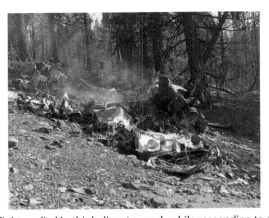

Fig. 11. Nine firefighters died in this helicopter crash while responding to a wildfire in 2008, Trinity County, CA. Other firefighters needed to be treated for psychological as well as physical injuries. (*Courtesy of* Larry Masterman, EMT-P, Medford, Oregon, Director of Emergency Services; Trinity County Sheriff's Office, Weaverville, CA.)

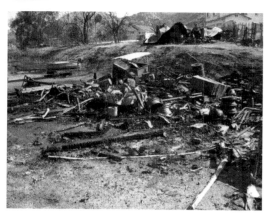

Fig. 12. Beginning to recover from the Pass Fire, Southern California, 2003. (*From* CAL FIRE. California Fire Siege of 2003: The story. Available at: http://www.fire.ca.gov/downloads/2003 FireStoryInternet.pdf. Accessed June 29, 2016.)

The distinction is important to nurses because of the impact on health and the number of people affected. Mid–twenty-first century projections show a large increase in the number of fires and property destruction leading, presumably, to increased health effects and cost (**Fig. 15, Table 3**).[15]

HEALTH IMPACTS OF WILDFIRES

Worldwide, approximately 339,000 people a year die from wildfire smoke, and billions are exposed as smoke travels over mountains, continents, and oceans.[29] Although the number and severity of wildfires are increasing in California and worldwide, not enough research has been conducted on the health effects of wildfires. Gaps in the literature include long-term sequelae from direct exposure to flames, heat, and toxic smoke and exposure to contaminated soil, water, and air after the fire.[4] Risk factors are increased for certain groups: vulnerable populations, such as the elderly; children; pregnant women; people with disabilities; those with preexisting conditions; and non-English speakers. Additional risk factors include the location of homes and ease of

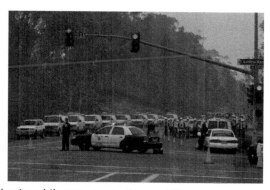

Fig. 13. Recovery begins while response continues. Utility crews prepare to restore power to affected communities during huge 2003 Southern California fires. (*From* CAL FIRE. California Fire Siege of 2003: The story. Available at: http://www.fire.ca.gov/downloads/2003 FireStory Internet.pdf. Accessed June 29, 2016.)

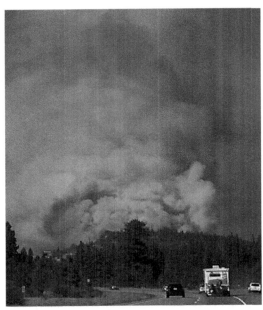

Fig. 14. Boles Fire, Weed, California, September 15, 2014. This summer fire was caused by an arsonist. Driven by strong winds, it destroyed one-third of the residences of the rural town of Weed, California, as well as other public and historic buildings. (*Courtesy of* Richard Hanes, NRP, EMT-P.)

access and egress of first responders and residents. Critical infrastructure is also a component of assessing risk: rural and less affluent areas have fewer resources on which to draw and are easily overwhelmed, whereas urban areas may be underfunded or have inadequate numbers or types of assets.[5,30]

Even less has been said about the hidden health costs related to wildfires. Richardson and colleagues[31] state, "human health impacts from exposure to wildfire smoke

Table 2 Wildfire characteristics and fuel sources, City of San Dimas, California		
Type	**Characteristics**	**Fuel**
Classic WUI fire	"Well-defined urban and suburban development presses up against open expanses of wild land areas."	• Hot, dry, windy weather • Fire resources inadequate to suppress or contain fire • Overwhelmed resources due to multiple fires • Large fuel load (ie, dense vegetation)
Mixed WUI fire	"Isolated homes, subdivisions, and small communities situated predominantly in wild land settings."	
Occluded WUI fire	"Islands of wild land vegetation occur inside a largely urbanized area."	

Adapted from City of San Dimas. Why are Wildfires a Threat to San Dimas? Available at: http://www.cityofsandimas.com/download.cfm?ID=3737.

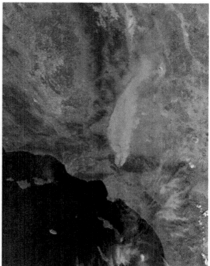

Santa Ana Fires	Summer Fires
Santiago Canyon Fire, October 22, 2007	Station Fire, August 29 , 2009

Fig. 15. Images of 2 types of California wildfires. Views are from the Southern California coast. The Santiago Canyon fire extended into Northern Mexico on the Baja Peninsula. The station fire was east of Los Angeles (large plume of smoke) with some other smaller fires in San Diego County. (*From* NASA earth observatory: NASA. NASA: California drought causing land to shrink. 2015. Available at: http://www.jpl.nasa.gov/news/news.php?feature 54693. Accessed March 18, 2016.)

Table 3
Comparison of types of California wildfires

Santa Ana wildfires	Non–Santa Ana (summer) wildfires
• September through December	• June through September
• Burn quickly and intensely	• Burn more slowly
• Shorter duration	• Longer duration
• Occur in wind corridors and more populated areas	• Occur in more remote inland areas, often at higher elevations
• More casualties	• Fewer casualties
• More property damage	• Less property damage
• Increased human and economic effects	• More competition for resources with other areas fighting summer fires
• Decreased humidity dries out vegetation; winds fan fires and cause secondary fires sometimes miles from original fire	• Interacts with summer heat and effects air quality
Projected Increase by 2050	
• Fires increase 64%	• Fires increase 77%
• Structures destroyed increase 20%	• Structures destroyed increase 90%

From Jin Y, Goulden ML, Faivre N, et al. Identification of two fire regimes in Southern California: implications for economic impact and future change. Extreme Mech Lett 2015;10:1–12.

are ignored in estimates of monetized damages from wildfires" and estimated the cost of illness from exposure to a large wildfire in Los Angeles at $9.50 per exposed person per day. The cost of just one wildfire-related health symptom was calculated at $84.42 per person per symptom. The investigators contend that current measures for calculating health costs vastly underestimate the actual costs.[31] In Southern California, with a population exceeding 22 million people, the cost of even a portion of people exposed to wildfire smoke is staggering.

Psychological effects can also be profound. An Australian study revealed that 12 months after the wildfire, 42% of patients requesting medical assistance were "potential psychiatric cases" whereas after the 2003 wildfires in California, of 357 patients seeking health care, 33% exhibited major depressive symptoms and 24% exhibited symptoms of posttraumatic stress disorder (PTSD). The effects of PTSD in children may extend into adulthood. Extensive media coverage can cause "vicarious traumatization," leading to PTSD in some individuals (**Fig. 16**, **Table 4**).[4]

DISASTER PREPAREDNESS, NURSING, AND WILDFIRES

It is critical for nurses to understand the relationship between the stakeholders shown in **Fig. 17**. Public health, emergency management, and the health care delivery system work in concert to increase competency, capacity, and capability in all phases of disaster. Nurses need to be aware of differences in triage and treatment of patients in disasters. This may occur in a utilitarian practice context where, instead of focusing on and doing all that can be done for the individual, the care model shifts to doing the greatest good for the greatest number of people.[32] Triage shifts to caring for people with available resources based not only on the severity of their injury or illness but also on their survivability as well.[24] Planning for the care of vulnerable populations may be better accomplished using the functional model approach, which looks at people's ability to function and do things for themselves, instead of the medical model, which is based on illness and disease. This is pertinent, for example, in hospital evacuations where some very ill patients may be ambulatory whereas others with a lower

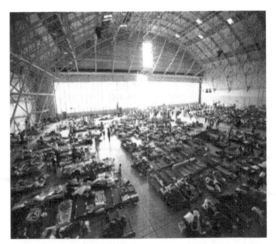

Fig. 16. More than 3000 evacuees in a shelter at Norton air force base during the 2003 Southern California wildfires. (*Photo by* Andrea Booher/FEMA News Photo-Location: San Bernardino, CA. Available at: www.fema.gov/media-library/assets/images/42220. Accessed April 1, 2016.)

Table 4 Major health effects of wildfires	
Direct health effects	
Exposure to flames and heat	• Burns • Death • Heat-induced illness • Other medical sequela
Toxic wildfire smoke	• Respiratory • Cardiovascular • Ocular • Short-term and-long term effects • Exposure to gases • Cancer • Potential lowered birthweights
Trauma	• Injuries due to falls, falling debris, etc. • Injuries and fatalities due to decreased visibility leading to traffic accidents • Electrical hazards • Tetanus • Other infections • Injuries due to animal encounters
Indirect health effects	
Psychological effects	• Panic • PTSD: survivors and responders • Grief and loss • Depression/somnolence • Anxiety • Hostility • Increased violence/domestic abuse • Increased smoking and drug use • Vicarious traumatization • Inability to focus/remember • Suicide
Pollution/contamination	• Contaminated soil • Contaminated water • Particulate matter in air • Carbon monoxide • Risk for contagious diseases • Agricultural hazards • Exposure to hazardous materials

Data from Refs.[2–4]

acuity may need more support.[33] Other considerations include staffing for those who cannot, or will not, come to work. Positions may need to be backfilled for those who leave to volunteer. Replacements are especially important for those who, for example, may be in home health/public/rural nursing and are the main contact for their patients (see **Fig. 17**).[30]

Nurses in Wildfire Situations

In 2003, wildfires devastated large areas of San Diego County. Hospitals were preparing for imminent evacuation of all patients. This was problematic; most hospitals have emergency surge plans but not plans for total evacuation.[1,5] In 2007, as wildfires again

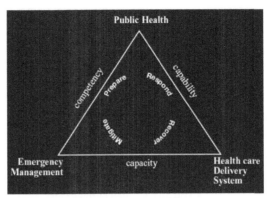

Fig. 17. The health emergency preparedness and response triad. (*From* USDA Agency for Healthcare Research and Quality. Available at: http://archive.ahrq.gov/news/ulp/btbriefs/brf8triad.htm. Accessed June 28, 2016.)

raged through northern San Diego County, the 109-bed Pomerado Hospital and Villa Pomerado, a 129-bed skilled nursing facility, activated their evacuation plans. These had been put in place after a hazard vulnerability assessment that identified wildfires and earthquakes as prime threats. Exercises with outside agencies are conducted twice yearly.[1] In contrast, the huge 2003 wildfires that burned 10% of San Diego County threatened 2 large hospitals that had to plan quickly for evacuation in a short period of time. Without a comprehensive evacuation plan, this challenged health care workers in numerous ways: (1) adjusting patient care for transporting in poor air quality; (2) preparing for hospital evacuation: increasing staff, discharging or transferring patients, arranging appropriate transportation, including helicoptering neonatal ICU patients to the Navy hospital ship USNS Mercy; (3) finding facilities to receive patients; and (4) personal challenges, including staff whose own homes and families were threatened (**Fig. 18**).[5]

Defining Nursing Roles

These examples indicate some of the important roles for nurses in wildfire disasters. Nurses in public health settings must shift focus to public health surge capacity and

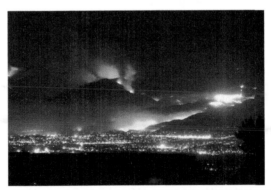

Fig. 18. Fires burning above San Diego, California, 2003. (*From* CAL FIRE. California Fire Siege of 2003: The story. Available at: http://www.fire.ca.gov/downloads/2003 FireStory Internet.pdf. Accessed June 29, 2016.)

population health, including that associated with facility evacuations.[34] Rural nurses have special roles given their limited resources and distance from outside support. In small, closely knit communities, rural nurses have multiple responsibilities and opportunities for input in the planning process, both in the community and in care facilities.[30] They can communicate with stakeholders and delineate roles and responsibilities. Another goal of preparedness specific to wildfires is to determine ways to minimize smoke exposure. The US Environmental Protection Agency (EPA) recommends providing Cleaner Air Shelters, where people at risk can go for respite from smoky air. These can be located in health care facilities or in public buildings meeting the EPA's criteria.[20,35] Hospitals may need to adjust ventilation systems and provide support for patients and staff should indoor air become smoky. In other areas, N95 masks or other personal protective equipment may need to be acquired.[30,34,35]

SUMMARY

Research is difficult in this emerging nursing specialty, partly because of the often sudden and chaotic nature of disasters. Consequently, there is little actual research on nursing and disasters. The challenges in disaster research are reflected in conducting research on wildfires and nursing. Other than anecdotal stories, little research is found in the literature. Disasters, including wildfires, do not happen within the timeframe of institutional review boards, so getting permission to conduct research is extremely difficult, even more so when vulnerable populations (a large percentage of people in disasters) are involved. Physical access to disaster sites and the ability to conduct research under tumultuous, fluid conditions are problematic as well. Institutions and their review boards need to develop criteria that enable researchers to conduct studies more nimbly while adhering to ethical principles, such as fidelity, nonmaleficence, and beneficence. According to the American Nurses Association *Code of Ethics for Nurses*, nurses must provide for the protection of human research participants and their rights of privacy and confidentiality (Provisions 3.1 and 3.2), and, at the same time, are obligated to contribute to the profession through "research and scholarly inquiry" as well as "developing, maintaining, and implementing professional practice standards" (Provisions 7.1 and 7.2).[36]

Kulig and colleagues have[30] conducted studies related to Canadian wildfires and rural nurses. As part of a multidisciplinary research team examining wildfires in rural communities, they identified challenges not only to rural nurses but also to all nurses in understanding what nurses need to do during wildfires and other disasters. They found that rural nurses who understand their communities and have theoretic knowledge of disaster nursing "potentially can reduce the impact of a disaster" and further recommended that "mentoring nursing students in disaster preparation and assisting in initiatives to address community recovery in the aftermath of a disaster" is a responsibility of all nurses.[30] Before nurses' roles in wildfires can by truly understood, all nurses must have a better overall knowledge of disasters and disaster nursing, beginning by using the International Council of Nurses Framework of Disaster Nursing Competencies to scaffold work and build knowledge.[22] From there, nurses will be better equipped to understand and prepare for what is needed in wildfire disasters.

REFERENCES

1. Barnett J, Dennis-Rouse M, Martinez V. Wildfire disaster leads to facilities evacuation. Orthop Nurs 2009;28(1):17–20.

2. Botey AP, Kulig JC. Family functioning following wildfires: recovering from the 2011 Slave Lake Fires. J Child Fam Stud 2014;23:1471–83.

3. Coppola DP. Introduction to international disaster management. 2nd edition. New York: Elsevier; 2011.

4. Finlay SE, Moffat A, Gazzard R, et al. Health impacts of wildfires. PLOS Curr Disasters 2012;1:1–27. Available at: http://currents.plos.org/disasters/article/health-impacts-of-wildfires/. Accessed March 16, 2016.

5. Hoyt KS, Gerhart AE. The San Diego wildfires: perspectives of healthcare. Disaster Management Response 2004;2(2):46–52.

6. Kieffer SW. Dynamics of disaster. New York: Norton; 2013.

7. Long S. Hospitals' wildfire emergency preparedness plans require communication and cooperation. Advance Healthcare Network for Nurses; 2008. Available at: http://nursing.advanceweb.com/Article/Planning-for-Californias-Wildfires.aspx. Accessed March 16, 2016.

8. Veneema TG, editor. Disaster nursing and emergency preparedness for chemical, biological, radiological, terrorism and other events. 2nd edition. New York: Springer; 2007.

9. NASA. NASA: California drought causing land to shrink. 2015. Available at: http://www.jpl.nasa.gov/news/news.php?feature=4693. Accessed March 18, 2016.

10. State of California. California drought. 2015. Available at: http://drought.ca.gov/. Accessed March 18, 2016.

11. Westerling AL, Cayan DR, Brown TJ, et al. Climate, Santa Ana winds, and autumn wildfires in Southern California. EOS 2004;85(31):289–300. Available at: http://ulmo.ucmerced.edu/pdffiles/04eos_westerling.pdf. Accessed March 18, 2016.

12. Corbett SW. Asthma exacerbations during a Santa Ana wind event in Southern California. Wilderness Environ Med 1996;4:306–11.

13. National Resources Defense Council. Climate change health threats in California. Available at: http://www.nrdc.org/health/climate/ca.asp. Accessed March 18, 2016.

14. California Department of Water Resources. Climate change. 2016. Available at: http://www.water.ca.gov/climatechange/. Accessed March 17, 2016.

15. Jin Y, Goulden ML, Faivre N, et al. Identification of two fire regimes in Southern California: Implications for economic impact and future change. Environ Res Lett 2015;10:1–12.

16. Azusa Pacific University Office of Institutional Research and Assessment. Fact sheet. Azusa (CA): Author; 2015. Available at: http://www.apu.edu/oira/factsheet/. Accessed March 17, 2016.

17. Citrus College. Citrus college factbook. Glendora (CA): Author; 2015. Available at: http://www.citruscollege.edu/admin/research/Documents/Fact%20Book/Spring2015FB.pdf. Accessed March 17, 2016.

18. Scauzillo S. Colby fire: firefighters say full containment possible by Sunday. San Gabriel Valley Tribune 2014. Available at: http://www.sgvtribune.com/general-news/20140117/colby-fire-firefighters-say-full-containment-possible-by-sunday#.VNKjkAhaX54.email. Accessed February 2, 2015.

19. Adelman DS, Legg TJ. Disaster nursing: a handbook for practice. Boston: Jones & Bartlett; 2009.

20. CalFire. California fire siege of 2003: the story. Available at: http://www.fire.ca.gov/downloads/2003FireStoryInternet.pdf. Accessed June 29, 2016.

21. Disease Prevention. What are the levels of disease prevention? 2013. Available at: http://www.diseaseprevention.com/what-are-the-levels-of-disease-prevention/. Accessed March 17, 2016.

22. International Council of Nurses. ICN framework of disaster nursing competencies. 2009. Available at: http://www.icn.ch/images/stories/documents/networks/DisasterPreparednessNetwork/Disaster_Nursing_Competencies_lite.pdf. Accessed March 17, 2016.

23. Warfield C. The disaster management cycle. Available at: http://www.gdrc.org/uem/disasters/1-dm_cycle.html. Accessed March 16, 2016.

24. National Disaster Life Support Foundation. Core disaster life support v.3.0. Augusta (GA): American Medical Association; 2010.

25. Williams J. Bushfire disaster: a rural nurse's perception. Aust Nurs J 2009;16(9):17.

26. Bushfire takes tool on nurses. Aust Nurs J 2009;16(8):5.

27. Sweet M. Nursing stories from the fires frontline. Aust Nurs J 2009;16(10):14.

28. CalFire. Incident information. 2013. Available at: http://cdfdata.fire.ca.gov/incidents/incidents_statsevents. Accessed March 18, 2016.

29. Loftis RL. Smoke from wildfires is killing hundreds of thousands of people. National Geographic 2015. Available at: http://news.nationalgeographic.com/2015/10/151029-wildfires-smoke-asthma-indonesia-california-health/. Accessed June 30, 2016.

30. Kulig JC, Edge D, Smolenski S. Wildfire disasters: Implications for rural nurses. Australas Nurs J 2014;17:126–34.

31. Richardson LA, Champ PA, Loomis JB. The hidden cost of wildfires: economic valuation of health effects of wildfire smoke exposure in Southern California. J For Econ 2012;18:14–35.

32. American Nurses Association (ANA). Adapting standards of care under extreme conditions. 2008. Available at: http://nursingworld.org/MainMenuCategories/WorkplaceSafety/Healthy-Work-Environment/DPR/TheLawEthicsofDisasterResponse/AdaptingStandardsofCare.pdf. Accessed March 31, 2016.

33. Reilly MJ, Markenson DS. Healthcare emergency management principles and practice. Boston: Jones and Bartlett; 2010.

34. California Association of Health Facilities. The San Diego model—A skilled nursing disaster preparedness and response plan. 2009. Available at: http://www.cahfdownload.com/cahf/dpp/SDModel-Final-08-27-09.pdf. Accessed March 17, 2016.

35. US Environmental Protection Agency. Wildfire smoke: a guide for public health officials. 2016. Available at: https://www3.epa.gov/airnow/wildfire_may2016.pdf. Accessed June 29, 2016.

36. American Nurses Association (ANA). Code of ethics for nurses with interpretive statements. Silver Springs (MD): American Nurses Association; 2015.

Evolution of a Nursing Model for Identifying Client Needs in a Disaster Shelter

A Case Study with the American Red Cross

Janice Springer, DNP, RN, PHN*, Mary Casey-Lockyer, RN, MHS, CCRN

KEYWORDS

- Disaster shelters • At-risk populations • Nursing care • Access and functional needs

KEY POINTS

- American Red Cross history goes back to Clara Barton and her work established a partnership with public health.
- Hurricane Katrina, presidential policy directives, and changes in the Federal Emergency Management Agency created an environment that encouraged a focus on disaster shelters and at-risk populations.
- When populations are either traumatically or deliberately evacuated and seek shelter, a system needs to be in place to receive them and assist in identifying their access and functional support needs.
- Studies show that people may not identify or recognize health or support needs for many hours or days after evacuation; there are more needs than might be predicted using census data.
- Registered nurses (RNs) have preparation across the age, gender, health, and illness continuum. An RN-led model of care is best positioned within a community health nursing framework to support and advocate for shelter populations.

INTRODUCTION

With a history of more than 100 years in disaster response, the American Red Cross has learned how to evolve. It has a mission to serve those in harms' way; has to be prepared to meet clients where they are; and must be prepared for the circumstances of the culture, geography, and demographics of the community in need that it is serving. This article showcases a process that began with the very roots of the American Red Cross, evolved through field experiences and literature review, was

Conflict of Interest: The authors have no conflict of interest in presenting this material.
American Red Cross, 2025 E St NW, Washington, DC 20006, USA
* Corresponding author.
E-mail address: Janice.Springer@redcross.org

scrutinized through an Institutional Review Board process, and ended with a product informed by nursing process and custom designed to reach all the clients who arrive in the throes of a disaster at a Red Cross shelter.

BACKGROUND

For nurses in the United States, the name Clara Barton and American Red Cross are forever linked. In many ways the story of Clara Barton is a beacon for the work that nurses do in modern times in disaster relief. She had a vision, she was an independent thinker, and she was determined to care for the underserved. Born in 1821, she was working at the US patent office in Washington DC when the civil war began. When she discovered that the Union Army had almost nothing prepared for medical care on the battlefield, she took up that cause and went into the fray. For the next several years she was determined to meet the needs of the soldiers, even turning down an opportunity to join the Army Nurses because women were not allowed into the battlefield. Although she was not a nurse by common definition of the time, she developed a solid reputation, bringing food, clothing, medical supplies, and whiskey, and delivering bedside care. She became known by one surgeon as "the true heroine of the age, the angel of the battlefield."[1]

After the war, recuperating in Europe, she met Henri Dunant, who had developed what later became the International Red Cross and the Geneva Conventions. His work inspired her to bring a version of the Red Cross to the United States and she spent the rest of her adult life working to have the Red Cross created. According to Kernodle,[2] author of *The Red Cross Nurse in Action 1882-1948*, Barton formed an association of Red Cross in 1881. During her lifetime she responded to many disasters, including the Johnstown floods of 1889.[2] After several disasters, military events, and persistence in her advocacy on behalf of the vulnerable affected by war and disaster, the United States Congress created a charter with the American Red Cross in 1905, including the expectation that the organization will "carry on a system of national and international relief in time of peace and to apply the same in mitigating the sufferings caused by pestilence, famine, fire, floods, and other great national calamities."[3] Kernodle[2] first mentions the creation of disaster shelters with nursing care after a tornado in Purvis, Mississippi, in 1908. Red Cross nursing evolved side by side with what became known as public health nursing. Mabel Boardman, an active and influential leader in Red Cross, worked with Lillian Wald, the founder of the Henry Street Settlement, and the two groups began to work together in the early years of the twentieth century.[2] This relationship ensured that Red Cross nursing and public health nursing were significantly aligned and had common goals around vulnerable populations. This theme is present and remains relevant into modern times in disaster preparedness and response.

KATRINA

The events of 9/11 stimulated much discussion and strategic planning for disasters, including Homeland Security Presidential Directive 5, which sought to enhance response to domestic events through establishing a single comprehensive national incident management system.[4] This directive started the process of creating systems for planning and response, but the events of Hurricane Katrina significantly changed the depth, pace, and faces of change.

Numerous articles were published post-Katrina that spoke to the needs for health care and to the profiles of vulnerable populations in shelters. A survey of shelters in the Houston area found disproportionate numbers of evacuees being of African

American origin, low income, without health insurance, and with chronic health conditions who were being managed in the New Orleans hospital system, which was now disabled or destroyed. Two other teams found similar results in Denver as Louisiana evacuees arrived there for housing and support.[5,6] More than 50% of their population had needs for health care, including refills of prescription medications, and nearly 50% had no health care insurance, an indicator for possible chronic lack of access to preventive care.

Dyer and colleagues[7] found a significant number of elderly in the Reliant Center, a disaster evacuation shelter in Houston post-Katrina. These were people who had no family, were so debilitated they could not advocate for themselves, and who could not avail themselves of services even within the shelter setting. Dr Dyer created a team with gerontology specialists to do a screening they called the Seniors Without Families Triage Tool (SWiFT) which was implemented by walking through the dormitory of the shelter, looking for seniors who seemed to be languishing or otherwise not able to attend to activities of daily living (ADLs). Jenkins and colleagues[8] had the unusual opportunity to review more than 31,000 health encounter records from across 8 states of post-Katrina shelters. There were no other (published) post-Katrina shelter client reviews this comprehensive. They found that the scope of health needs in a shelter were vast; from minor, such as a headache, to acute, such as a new respiratory illness; from preventive (63.8% of encounters) to extensive management of chronic health conditions, including referrals to clinics or hospitals for such events as chest pain or infection.

Judith Saunders, DNSc, CNS,[9] was deployed to a Red Cross–managed evacuation shelter in Jackson, Mississippi, after Katrina as a volunteer. To try to make some sense of the multitude of nursing and mental health care interventions they needed in order to keep that population as healthy and safe as they could, she used Flaskerud and Winslows'[10] theory of vulnerable populations. The model of vulnerable populations is a community health–based model that proposes that relative risk, resource availability, and health status are related. The theory demonstrates relationships between poverty and health, between socioeconomic status and health, and between personal choices in diet, exercise, and habits, and health. The 3 theoretic concepts described at the level of community are shown to affect the health of individuals.[10] The model has been used across multiple disciplines, including sociology, psychology, and public health (**Fig. 1**).

Case Study Katrina

In the early weeks after Katrina, the author was the lead registered nurse (RN) in a shelter that had more than 1800 residents. There were numerous opportunities to affect health through simple interventions. There were only about 16 sinks for hand washing. These were in the 4 bathrooms that were in the shelter. Porta Potties were outside, but no hand washing stations. We started an aggressive campaign of distribution of giant bottles of hand sanitizer. Hand sanitizing stations were set up within the shelter, at the health desk, at the entrance to the food consumption areas, in the serving line, near the toilet areas, and at most desks. One day a donation of pocket-sized hand sanitizers arrived and we put 1 on each pillow in the building. We had many infants on bottle feeding and were fortunate enough to have a side kitchen in the arena with a sterilizer installed. One nurse created a process and teaching guide and, with minimal supervision, the mothers quickly took over that area of responsibility and served very conscientiously.[11]

Almost immediately after Katrina, there was a swirl of controversies around shelter response, which came to the attention of the US Department of Health and Human

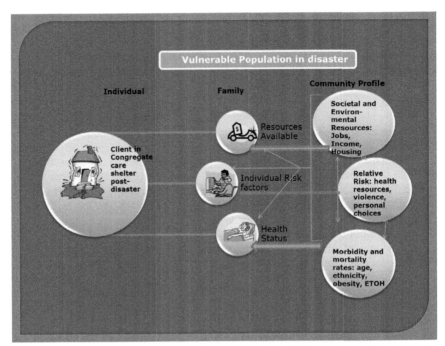

Fig. 1. Individual impact from disaster. There is a paucity of literature on disaster nursing practice. Of the more than 250 articles reviewed for this project a small handful of articles emerged out of nurses personal experiences after Hurricanes Katrina and Gustav. Two Nurses, Saunders and Missildine, one after Katrina and one after Hurricane Gustav, used Flaskerud and Winslow's[10] theory of vulnerable populations to frame their findings in disaster shelters. They defined vulnerable populations as social groups who have an increased relative risk or susceptibility to adverse health outcomes, including increased morbidity, mortality, and diminished quality of life. For the community profile, quality of life is influenced by (1) societal and environmental resources; (2) community health resources, violence, and personal choices; and (3) age, ethnicity, morbidity, and mortality. The individual and family unit resources in place when disaster strikes, and on the left is what happens to individuals who arrive in a shelter after or as a disaster strikes. Every person in that shelter is disconnected from their routines and resources and is at risk of becoming vulnerable. Flaskerud and Winslow's[10] conceptual model of vulnerable populations emphasizes the responsibility of the community to provide resources to achieve health goals and reduce risk for vulnerable populations. Their model is used across multiple disciplines, including sociology, psychology, and public health. This theory provided the backdrop to inform analysis of the needs of clients in shelters. (*Courtesy of* Janice Springer, DNP, RN, PHN, Foley, MN; and *From* Flaskerud J, Winslow B. Conceptualizing vulnerable populations' health-related research. Nurs Res 1998;47(2);69–78.)

Services (HHS) and the American Red Cross. These two groups began to work immediately on a shelter intake screening tool that was released as a joint effort in 2006.[12] This tool was disseminated primarily throughout the Red Cross sheltering system with an expectation for it to be used as clients arrived at the shelter to determine whether they had health, mental health, access, or functional support needs. Access and functional need support is particularly oriented to identify persons with disabilities, persons with caregivers, and others in the population who may need assistance to maintain their independence within the shelter environment.

Over 3 years, the author and others tried to use this instrument to have early identification of clients who may need assistance, but there were many barriers to its use. During a flood event in Fargo, North Dakota, in 2009, the author had sufficient staff to organize a system to critically manage the use and analysis of this intake tool. In a review of more than 200 screened clients in shelters, it was clear that those asking the questions of the clients did not understand the questions, the clients did not understand the purpose of the questions, and the expectation that having answers to the questions would somehow clarify whether the client would be best accommodated in that shelter were all in error.[13]

EVOLUTION OF A NEW SCREENING TOOL

At the same time these data were being shared with Red Cross disaster leadership, the Federal Emergency Management Agency released a new document to guide shelters: *Guidance on Planning for Integration of Functional Needs Support Services in General Population Shelters.*[14] This document arose out of multiple complaints to the Department of Justice and others indicating a clear pattern around persons with disabilities being excluded from or not being supported in general populations shelters.

In 2010, a workgroup formed of multiple stakeholders, including FEMA's Office of Disability Integration and Coordination (ODIC), the US Department of Health and Human Services Offices of Emergency Preparedness under the Assistant Secretary for Preparedness and Response, the American Red Cross, several supporting groups such as the Agency on Aging and At-Risk Individuals, Behavioral Health and Community Resilience (ABC), also from HHS. Over 2 years this workgroup coordinated with the authors (as team leaders) in support of a study to investigate better ways to identify clients early in their arrival to the shelters and to change the culture of sheltering to be more aware of the tenets of the Americans with Disabilities Act to expect inclusion, self-determination, and accommodation.[15]

Along this pathway, several things were learned that informed the evolution of the new system. First, that the original form designed in 2006 was based on a premise, likely unspoken, that persons arrive at a shelter with something like a chief complaint. A medical model presumes that, if you just ask the right question, you will get the answer you need in order to decide what to do next. Over this time period, 2 additional styles of intake screening forms were used on shelter populations to try to establish the clients' needs and, consistently, the clients did not know what we were trying to get at. They did not answer Yes/No to Yes/No-style questions, they told their story. When a persons' diagnosis was revealed, it did not help determine what functional support needs the client might have had. For example, if someone claims to have chronic obstructive pulmonary disease, this may give a hint of what the person might need, but not whether that person can sleep lying flat on a cot, has all the needed medications, needs to use oxygen, and so forth. In one situation, the local public health department went to a Red Cross shelter during Hurricane Ike, reviewed the clients there, and sent a list to the lead of the Red Cross health team of who needed to be moved and why. Every reason was a diagnosis, which gave no clue to what supportive needs were not being met. A person who uses a wheelchair for mobility should be accommodated in the general population shelter, not moved because they have a diagnosis of a musculoskeletal condition.

System problems were identified as well. The original premise was that these questions could be asked by registration clerks as part of the shelter registration process. Over several disaster relief operations it was noted that the registration staff did not do them or did so with great reluctance. Interviews showed that they were afraid of what to do with a "Yes" (I have needs) answer; were not comfortable receiving what might be considered private health information; and felt too pressured with the job of registration to have the additional duty of intake screening. During the Fargo event, there were enough RN staff deployed for an RN to be assigned to every registration desk for the sole purpose of doing the screening. This arrangement freed registration staff to fulfill their role, and also put the clients with interviewers who had experience with personal health needs, and who could immediately intervene to assist if needed.

As the multiagency workgroup proceeded to review the outcomes of the tools, and it became clear that the screening to identify access and functional, health, and mental health needs was perhaps better under the umbrella of the Health Services staff, where only licensed health providers are assigned, there was push-back from the disability community. The ODIC, representing the disability community in general, pointed out that there is a long history of persons with disabilities being treated as medical problems to be solved, not as persons first. Putting the screening process under the umbrella of health services and licensed health care providers seemed familiar in uncomfortable ways. Through several discussions of explaining that disaster shelter nursing is public health nursing, and that principles of public health practice are all about supporting individuals within their environment, inclusion, self-determination, and independence, the value of moving the screening process to what became a 2-step model was clarified.

In public health parlance, when persons are evacuated because of a disaster, either before an event or after, they have become at risk or vulnerable. The disability community is not comfortable being labeled as either (Marcie Roth, personal communications, 2011). However, public health nurses, in their role in disaster shelters, are perfectly poised both to support the independence of the population in the shelter and to have the awareness and understanding of resources when the circumstances of the disaster or living in the shelter environment contribute to people not being able to fully care for themselves.[9]

The synthesis of all the field experiences and conversations became crystallized during a hurricane event in North Carolina shelters.

During Hurricane Irene, 3 shelters were staffed with nurses who had been directed to implement a new trial screening tool and to systematically ensure that every family unit was screened. Because of the storm and the logistics, 1 team of nurses arrived at the shelter that had been open for 3 days. The staff there had done some random screening at registration, but nothing formal. As the nurses made the rounds, using a new interview tool, interesting things began to unfold. Once again, it was revealed that the content of the questions was not necessarily leading to the anticipated answers. The questions became the platform for allowing a conversation between the nurses and the shelter clients. Within the conversations and the relationship came the information to guide support of health, mental health, access, and functional support needs. Several scenarios revealed that even though persons may have been asked about having needs when they arrived, it was the nurses who had the knowledge and skill set to ask the questions that were not on the form. One woman was having some trouble getting enough oxygen to breath. She was weak, had dusky coloring, and had to pause between sentences as she was being interviewed. To the nurse's inquiries she replied: "Yes, I am having a little trouble breathing; yes, I have a concentrator; well, yes, it is here in the trunk of my car." For 3 days she had been without her necessary equipment because no one thought to ask her, and, as she admitted, she "did not want to bother anyone."[15]

Building caring relationships, grounded in social justice, focused on the health of entire populations, in this case the shelter population, all are part of what is known as the cornerstones of public health nursing.[16] In the time of Clara Barton, Mable Boardman, and Lillian Wald, nurses in disaster response were practicing public health nursing. This awareness was added to the cumulative knowledge of 3 years of study and a new system for identifying access and functional, health, and mental health needs of clients in shelters was developed (**Box 1**).

SYSTEM REDESIGN: INTAKE, COT-TO-COT AND CMIST

In Hurricane Irene and other events, we continued to find that many clients were simply not aware of their needs for even the first 3 to 4 days after evacuation, even though the population in a general shelter is typically persons who have come from home. They may be able to identify urgent needs on arrival at the shelter, so it was important to maintain at least some level of early opportunity for self-identification of needs. The system has 2 phases, and is organized to ensure that clients have multiple opportunities to share their needs with staff in a private and safe setting, and at the time they are able.

Phase 1 is called Registration Intake and is a strategy of 2 observations and 2 questions made at the registration intake desk, which can be done by nonlicensed health care providers, or anyone working at that desk (**Fig. 2**). The observations are to reinforce what people do naturally, but with guidance for ways to engage with clients who are clearly upset, or who may have a disability or support need. The 2 observations are written down, because even though it may seem obvious that you are observing the clients as they come through the door, the circumstances of this kind of situation require concrete and easily repeatable steps. Predeployment training for this particular job is sometimes minimal, and to ensure that every worker has the same base it is supported by having it all written down. The 2 questions are designed to offer immediate opportunity for sharing needs, to help clients start to think about what they might have forgotten in evacuation. The questions were constructed based on the principles that persons under stress need short sentences and concrete directions and time frames.[17]

Box 1
Cornerstones of public health nursing

Public health nursing practice:

- Focuses on the health of entire populations

- Reflects community priorities and needs

- Establishes caring relationships with communities, systems, individuals, and families

- Grounded in social justice, compassion, sensitivity to diversity, and respect for the worth of all people, especially the vulnerable

- Encompasses mental, physical, emotional, social, spiritual, and environmental aspects of health

- Promotes health through strategies driven by epidemiologic evidence

- Collaborates with community resources to achieve those strategies, but can and will work alone if necessary

- Derives its authority for independent action from the Nurse Practice Act

Data from Minnesota Department of Health. Cornerstones of public health nursing. 2007. Available at: http://www.health.state.mn.us/divs/opi/cd/phn/docs/0710phn_cornerstones.pdf. Accessed November 12, 2011.

Registration Intake

These are yes/no observations and questions to support registration staff in identifying and obtaining assistance and supplies for shelter residents.

Observations

1. Does the client or a family member appear to be in need of immediate medical attention, appear too overwhelmed or agitated to complete registration, or is a threat to themselves or others?   **Yes** ☐   **No** ☐

> *If Yes, STOP the registration process and do one of the following:*
> - *If situation is critical and no support is available, call 911 if available.*
> - *Contact Health Services and/or Mental Health worker on site.*
> - *If no health or mental health resource on site, direct concern to Shelter Manager, or*
>
> *If NO, continue the registration process.*

2. If the client has a service animal, uses a wheelchair/walker or demonstrates any other circumstance where it appears they may need help in the shelter, acknowledge their need and offer assistance this may include contacting a health services worker.

> *Contact Shelter Manager for additional support when needed.*

Questions:

1. Is there anything you or a member of your family needs right now to stay healthy while in the shelter?   **Yes** ☐   **No** ☐   If NO, is there anything you will need in the next 6–8 h ? **Yes** ☐ **No** ☐

2. Do you/family member have a health, mental health, disability, or other condition about which you are concerned? ☐ **Yes** ☐ **No**

> *If question #1, or #2 has a YES answer, Health Services and/or Mental Health services must be notified.*
>
> *Priorities:*
>
> **First:** *Contact Health or Mental Health Services worker on site;*
>
> *OR if no health or mental health on site,*
>
> **Second:** *Contact Shelter Manager for follow-up*
>
> *OR*
>
> **Third:** *Make a list of clients who have a "yes" response and give the list to the health services volunteer when they arrive.*

Fig. 2. Phase 1 registration intake. (*Data from* American Red Cross. Registration intake tool. 2015. Available at:http://www.nationalmasscarestrategy.org/wp-content/uploads/2015/07/Red-Cross-Registration-Intake-Form-051613.pdf. Accessed April 4, 2016; with permission.)

Each of the observations and questions sections has a triage strategy so that, if a clerk is left with a question about how to handle a situation, the decision tree is on the same form. This version is the final form adopted by the American Red Cross.[18]

Phase 2 reflects an evolution of Dyer and colleagues'[7] work combined with principles of management by walking around and key elements of assessment and relationship building by the nurses.[7,19] It is called Cot-to-Cot. After the first offer of needs identification at registration, it was observed repeatedly that clients need multiple opportunities to reveal their needs. They need to be confident that their intimate requests will be managed with confidentiality, and they need to recognize it themselves; it is sometimes hours to days before clients recognize that they have pain, have forgotten a medication, or will soon run out of consumable medical supplies such as catheters or colostomy bags. In addition to having a health desk where clients can self-present with requests for assistance, nurses need to make rounds on a regular basis.

Cot-to-Cot is the physical event of being deliberate about checking in with individuals and families. It can also be used as a metaphor for population assessment, a strategy for maintaining an awareness of the mental health of the population and individuals, and a method for building the trust relationship so crucial for vulnerable groups to feel comfortable with sharing. Making rounds through Cot-to-Cot is being visible, and a way to set the tone that the shelter staff in general and the health care and mental health care staff in particular are concerned about clients' well-being.

Cot-to-Cot also contributes to surveillance. A fundamental part of public health nursing is population surveillance. In a shelter population, because of circumstances before or during evacuation, and/or consequences of congregate living, there may be high risk of disease or injury. Daily surveillance is crucial to staying ahead of circumstances that might need intervention.[20] In addition to nurses gathering data from self-presentations to the health desk, with chief complaints or other requests, observations made through Cot-to-Cot over several shifts and days allow the staff to recognize other patterns that may not be evident through individual requests for assistance.

For example, during routine Cot-to-Cot rounds in a shelter in North Carolina after Hurricane Irene, the RN noticed that staff and shelter residents were having trouble with 1 particular teenager. The teen and his mother were also distressed. Further investigation determined that the boy was autistic and needed a different sleeping environment and some options for areas with less stimulation, such as lower lights and less noise. The nurse advocated for different sleeping arrangements, then did an in-service on autism for staff and later for residents, making a safer environment for all.

Every 10 years, the US Census Bureau sends or brings a set of questions to every household. Persons may self-identify as being disabled, being hard of hearing, with low-vision, or a variety of other conditions.[21] One way to anticipate the percentage of a local population that might come to the shelter with access and functional support needs is to use local county census data. During 2 studies (**Fig. 3**), 1 shelter in a tornado and, later, during Hurricane Irene in North Carolina, 4 shelters from 4 different counties were compared for access and functional support needs identified compared with census data for the percentage of the population in that county who self-identified as having a disability.

In 3 of the 4 shelters, the percentage of persons with needs was higher than might have been predicted by using census data. A broader and more inclusive perspective is needed.

Cot-to-Cot provides a nurse-led methodology to maximize the effectiveness of nurses and other licensed care providers in disaster shelters. However, our studies showed that a framework of language was needed to consider a more inclusive view than the medical and even ADL model provides.

Over the years, 4 different interview screening tools were tested, and none seemed to meet the need. The multiagency team considered, "could the CMIST model inform our content?" CMIST is an acronym for communication, maintaining health, independence, services, support and self-determination, and transportation.[22] Our studies showed that traditional interview questions were not establishing our clients' needs. We needed to move away from a diagnosis-based system into a broader view that encompassed health, mental health, access, and functional needs, and with an eye to population health (**Fig. 4**). The CMIST instrument as used by the American Red Cross is not designed as an interview but as a set of suggestions about various items that might need to be considered in reaching out to offer assistance. It is broader than

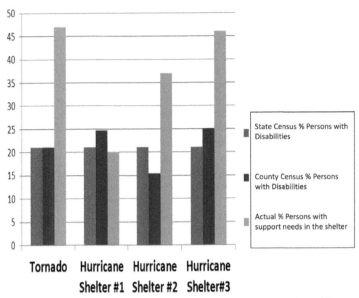

Fig. 3. Comparison of shelter persons with needs versus state census data. (*Courtesy of* Janice Springer, DNP, RN, PHN, Foley, MN.)

ADL's, includes health and mental health data, and considers multiple strategies to support maintaining independence in the shelter environment.

In 2012, CMIST was tested during Hurricane Sandy. Over approximately 1 week, nurses in American Red Cross shelters did CMIST assessments in 17 shelters in the Long Island area (**Fig. 5**). The author reviewed data that included 1035 individuals. The distribution showed that approximately 70% of the needs were under Maintaining Health and included such items as dietary support (41 persons), medication refills (74 persons), and wound management support needs. Transportation was a major need in 1 shelter on Staten Island, because most people did not own cars, and the subway system was broken at their end of the line. Communication was mostly needs for translators, but later in the response we needed to find and replace a screen reader for a vision-impaired client whose reader was lost in the storm.

The system is in place and being refined. However, a larger question looms, for Red Cross and for the future. How can a workforce of nurses be engaged and prepared to meet the ongoing needs of disasters?

SUMMARY: CHALLENGES GOING FORWARD FOR A TRAINED NURSING WORKFORCE

In the Pacific Northwest, a zone called Cascadia is predicted to have a massive earthquake with consequent tsunami, potentially destroying large parts of Oregon and Washington State.[23] In the central part of the United States the New Madrid Fault creates a potential for a catastrophic earthquake event. This area had a massive earthquake in 1811 and is predicted to have another in modern times.[24] The planning documents for this event, which would affect 4 states significantly and 8 states to some extent, include predictions for:

710,000 buildings destroyed
42,000 search and rescue personnel working in 1500 teams
3500 damaged bridges

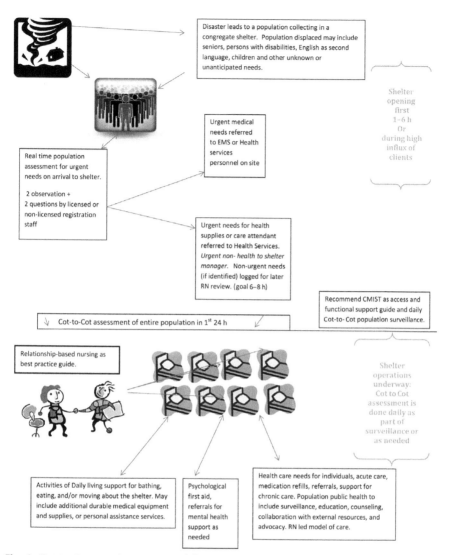

Fig. 4. Cot-to-Cot meeting access and functional needs in mass care shelters. (*Courtesy of* Janice Springer, DNP, RN, PHN, Foley, MN.)

2.6 million households without power
86,000 injuries and fatalities
130 damaged hospitals
7.2 million people displaced, with 2 million people seeking shelter

In addition to the daily disasters of floods, hurricanes, wildfires, and human-made hazards such as oil spills and transportation accidents, where will the trained volunteers come from for these catastrophic events? How will health care be provided in shelters for 2 million displaced persons?

In October of 2015, the Kaiser Family Foundation showed that there were 3.9 million professionally active nurses in the United States.[25] This number represents by far the largest block of trained health care personnel in the country. Baack and Alfred[26]

CMIST Worksheet	Total number of family included on this form _____.

DATE:	CLIENT/FAMILY NAME:	COUNTY/STATE:
Client location in shelter:		Interviewer:

This is a document to cover possible considerations for scenarios of access and functional needs. This is not an all-inclusive checklist, but rather serves as a simple guideline for referral purposes.

COMMUNICATION

NEED:	ACTION:
☐ Access to auxiliary communication service	☐ Provide written materials in alternative format (Braille, large and high contrast print, audio recording, or readers) ☐ Provide visual public announcements ☐ Provide qualified sign language or oral interpreter ☐ Provide qualified foreign language interpreter
☐ Access to auxiliary communication device	☐ Provide access to teletypewriter [TTY, TDD, or CapTel] or cell phone with texting capabilities; pen and paper.
☐ Replacement of auxiliary communication equipment	☐ Provide replacement eyeglasses ☐ Provide replacement hearing aid and/or batteries

MAINTAINING HEALTH

NEED:	ACTION:
☐ Special diet ☐ Food Allergies_____(type)	☐ Provide alternative (low sugar, low sodium, pureed, gluten-free, dairy-free, peanut-free) food and beverages; _____(diet type)
☐ Medical supplies and/or equipment for every day care (including medications) *not* related to mobility *For replacement eyeglasses or hearing aid, see Communication* *For assistive mobility equipment (e.g., wheelchair), see Independence*	***Refer to Disaster Health Services** to provide or procure one or more of the following:* ☐ Replacement medication ☐ Wound management/dressing supplies ☐ Diabetes management supplies (e.g., test strips, lances, syringes) ☐ Bowel or bladder management supplies (e.g., colostomy supplies, catheters) ☐ Oxygen supplies and/or equipment
☐ Assistance with medical care normally provided in the home setting ☐ Allergies (environmental or other high risk)_____(type) *For medical treatments that are **not** normally provided in the home setting (e.g., dialysis), see Transportation*	***Refer to Disaster Health Services** to provide assistance with one or more of the following:* ☐ Administration of medication ☐ Storage of medication (e.g., refrigeration) ☐ Wound management ☐ Bowel or bladder management ☐ Use of medical equipment ☐ Universal precautions and infection prevention and control (e.g., disposal of bio-hazard materials, such as needles in sharps containers)
☐ Support for pregnant women ☐ Support for nursing mothers; ☐ Infant care availability	☐ Provide support by ongoing observation ☐ Provide support and/or room for breastfeeding women ☐ Assure diaper changing area is available
☐ Access to a quiet area	☐ Provide access to a quiet room or space within the shelter (e.g., for elderly persons, people with psychiatric disabilities, parents with very young children, children and adults with autism)
☐ Access to a temperature-controlled area	☐ Provide access to an air-conditioned and/or heated environment (e.g., for those who cannot regulate body temperature)
☐ Mental health care (e.g., anxiety and stress management)	☐ ***Refer to Disaster Mental Health Services***

Fig. 5. Red Cross CMIST Worksheet. (*Data from* American Red Cross. CMIST worksheet. Available at: http://www.maphn.org/Resources/Documents/CMIST%20WORKSHEET%20FINAL.pdf. Accessed April 4, 2016; with permission.)

surveyed 620 nurses asking how well prepared they thought they were to respond to a disaster. Most nurses reported a perception of low to average competence in responding to a major disaster event. In general, they found that the best strategy for preparing nurses to be confident in responding to a disaster was their prior experience of having

CMIST Worksheet   **Total number of family included on this form _____.**

INDEPENDENCE	
NEED:	**ACTION:**
☐ Durable medical equipment for individuals with conditions that affect mobility	☐ Provide assistive mobility equipment (e.g., wheelchair, walker, cane, crutches)
	☐ Provide assistive equipment for bathing and/or toileting (e.g., raised toilet seat with grab bars, handled shower, bath bench)
	☐ Provide accessible cot (may be a crib, inclined head or other bed type)
☐ Power source to charge battery-powered assistive devices	☐ Provide power source to charge battery-powered assistive devices
☐ Bariatric accommodations	☐ Provide bariatric cot or bed
☐ Service animal accommodations	☐ Provide area where service animal can be housed, exercised, and toileted
	☐ Provide food and supplies for service animal
☐ Infant supplies and/or equipment	☐ Provide infant supplies (e.g., formula, baby food, diapers, crib)

SERVICES, SUPPORT AND SELF-DETERMINATION	
NEED:	**ACTION:**
☐ Adult personal assistance services	☐ Identify family member or friend caregiver
☐ Child personal assistance services	☐ Assign qualified shelter volunteer to provide personal assistance services
*Incl. general observation and/or assistance with **non-medical** activities of daily living, such as grooming, eating, bathing, toileting, dressing and undressing, walking, etc.*	☐ Contact local agency to provide personal assistance services
	☐ Coordinate childcare support such as play areas; age-appropriate activities; equal access to resources.

TRANSPORTATION	
NEED:	**ACTION:**
☐ Transportation to designated facility for medical care or treatment	☐ Coordinate provision of accessible shelter vehicle and driver for transportation
☐ Transportation for non-medical appointment	☐ Contact local transit service to provide accessible transportation

Actions:

☐ No needs identified
☐ Contact Shelter Manager
☐ Contact Disaster Mental Health Services
☐ Agency, *please provide agency name*

☐Other_____

Followup/Resolution/date_____

_____

Disaster Health Services print name/signature/date_____

Fig. 5. (*continued*)

responded. The American Red Cross manages an average of 60% of the shelters operating in the country.[27] Their workforce is almost entirely voluntary, and funding is primarily through donations. Estimates of nurses trained and ready to respond were more than 100,000 nurses serving through the Red Cross during WWII. From their publication *The Changing Face of Help*, the Red Cross reports that "nearly every American family had a Red Cross connection either receiving aid or, in the case of their 7.5 million volunteers, delivering aid."[28] As of 2015, that trained workforce is about 15,000 nurses and other licensed health providers.[27] The Medical Reserve Corps was instituted after Presidential Policy Directive 5 for local (not deployable) response, and is funded through grants from the Federal Government and local authorities. The mission of the Medical Reserve Corps is to establish teams of local volunteer medical and public health professionals who can contribute their skills and expertise throughout the year and during times of community need. The corps has 987 community-based units in 50 states and a role in providing public health surge.[29]

Through their public health capabilities framework, public health departments have been encouraged to work with partners to develop the depth and breadth of preparedness needed to respond to local disasters.[30] For the United States to sustain a catastrophic event, all nurses will need to contribute to the response. There is a need for health care providers to be trained in disaster relief and to affiliate with an umbrella organization for maximum regional readiness.[31]

Registration Intake, Cot-to-Cot, and CMIST are used within the RN-led model of care for American Red Cross disaster shelters. The RN-led model was created through the Blueprint for Action,[32] to align Red Cross nursing with the Institute of Medicine collaboration *The Future of Nursing: Leading Change, Advancing Health*.[33] The language of Cot-to-Cot and CMIST help move the knowledge, skills and abilities nurses bring to the clients impacted by disaster, toward promotion of self-determination through "assisting clients to identify their needs".

The disasters of 2015 provided opportunities for testing the strength of the model in early identification of clients in shelters with health care and functional support needs. One RN, John Decker, who was part of the original study in North Carolina in 2011, returned to floods in South Carolina in 2015. He said that doing the Cot-to-Cot has become a natural and automatic process of working in the shelter. As a manager in that disaster, with multiple shelters opening in rapid succession, he was able to adapt the model in a new way as a rapid assessment team concept. He could send a small team to the new shelter and have them do a Cot-to-Cot survey, with CMIST in hand, and get a snapshot of the needs in that shelter. His team then taught these concepts to the shelter team, already on site, supporting them to be able to survey the clients as they arrived and secure early support for meeting their needs.

Nurses bring a unique skill set to those affected by disaster. Nurses are committed advocates for their clients; educated to provide clinical services, surveillance, education, and referrals; and driven to prevent illness and promote healthy communities. RNs have preparation across the age, gender, health, and illness continuum. An RN-led model of care is best positioned within a community health nursing framework to support and advocate for shelter populations. The more nurses prepared for disaster response, the better the communities will survive and recover from them.

For more information about nursing and volunteering with the American Red Cross, go to www.redcross.org.

REFERENCES

1. Oates S. A woman of valor: Clara Barton and the civil war. New York: The Free Press; 1994.
2. Kernodle P. The Red Cross nurse in action 1882-1948. New York: Harper and Brothers; 1949.
3. American Red Cross. Congressional charter, 1905. 2015. Available at: www.redcross.orgabout-us/history/federal-charter. Accessed December 3, 2015.
4. Presidential Directive 5. Department of Homeland Security. 2003. Available at: www.dhs.gov. Accessed December 3, 2015.

5. Brodie M, Weltzien E, Altman D, et al. Experiences of Hurricane Katrina evacuees in Houston shelters: implications for future planning. Am J Public Health 2008; 96(8):1402–8.

6. Ghosh T, Patnaik J, Vogt R. Rapid needs assessment among Hurricane Katrina evacuees in Metro-Denver. J Health Care Poor Underserved 2007;18:362–8.

7. Dyer C, Regev M, Burnett J, et al. SWiFT: a rapid triage tool for vulnerable older adults in disaster situations. Disaster Med Public Health Prep 2008; 2(Suppl 1):S45.

8. Jenkins J, McCarthy M, Kelen G, et al. Changes needed in the care for sheltered persons: a multistate analysis from Hurricane Katrina. Am J Disaster Med 2009; 4(2):101–6.

9. Saunders J. Vulnerable populations in an American Red Cross shelter after Hurricane Katrina. Perspect Psychiatr Care 2007;43(1):30–7.

10. Flaskerud J, Winslow B. Conceptualizing vulnerable populations' health-related research. Nurs Res 1998;47(2):69–78.

11. Springer J. Public Health in a Katrina shelter. In: Veenema TG, editor. Disaster nursing and emergency preparedness for chemical, biological and radiological terrorism and other hazards. 2nd edition. New York: Springer; 2007. p. 201–2.

12. Dodgen D, Shea M, Wood A. Initial intake and assessment tool presented by the U.S. Department of Health and Human Services and The American Red Cross at 2009 Integrated Training Summit. 2015. Available at: http://www.integratedtrainingsummit. org/presentations/2009/weekend_workshops/i_-_orientation_to_the_american_ red_cross_shelter_intake_and_assessment_tool_-_dodgen.pdf. Accessed October 23, 2014.

13. Springer J, West J, Cunningham D. Initial intake and assessment tool poster session. American Red Cross Leadership Seminar. 2010.

14. Guidance on planning for integration of functional needs support services in general populations shelters. FEMA; 2010. Available at: http://www.fema.gov/pdf/ about/odic/fnss_guidance.pdf. Retrieved August, 2015.

15. Springer J. A cot-to-cot model for meeting client needs in disaster shelters [dissertation]. University of Minnesota, School of Nursing; 2012.

16. Minnesota Department of Health. Cornerstones of public health nursing. 2007. Available at: http://www.health.state.mn.us/divs/opi/cd/phn/docs/0710phn_ cornerstones.pdf. Accessed November 12, 2011.

17. Schwarz N, Oyserman D. Asking questions about behavior: cognition, communication and questionnaire construction. Am J Eval 2001;22(2):127–60.

18. American Red Cross. Registration intake tool. 2015. Available at: http://www. nationalmasscarestrategy.org/wp-content/uploads/2015/07/Red-Cross-Registration- Intake-Form-051613.pdf. Accessed April 4, 2016.

19. Peters T, Waterman R. In search of excellence. New York: Harper Collins; 1982.

20. Centers for Disease Control and Prevention. Surveillance in Hurricane Evacuation centers–Louisiana, September-October 2005. MMWR Morb Mortal Wkly Rep 2006;55(2):32–5.

21. US Census Bureau. Census 2010. 2011. Available at: http://2010.census.gov/ 2010census/about/. Accessed November 12, 2011.

22. Kailes JI, Enders A. Moving beyond "special needs:" A framework for emergency management and planning. Journal of Disability Policy Studies 2007; 17(4):230.

23. Goldfinger C, Nelson CH, Morey AE, et al. Turbidite event history—Methods and implications for Holocene paleoseismicity of the Cascadia subduction zone: U.S.

Geological Survey Professional Paper 1661–F, 170 p, 64. 2012. Available at: http://pubs.usgs.gov/pp/pp1661/f www.mae.ccc.illinois.edu. Accessed December 3, 2015.

24. Mid-America Earthquake Center. Impact of new Madrid seismic zone earthquakes on the central USA. Urbana (IL): University of Illinois; 2009.

25. Kaiser Family Foundation. Total number of professionally active nurses. Available at: www.kff.org. Accessed October 23, 2015.

26. Baack S, Alfred D. Nurses' perception and perceived competence in managing disasters. J Nurs Scholarsh 2013;45(3):281–7 [Wiley Company, Hoboken (NJ)].

27. American Red Cross. Red Cross nursing (n.d.). Available at: www.redcross.org. Accessed November 14, 2015.

28. American Red Cross Turns 125. The changing face of help. Cleveland (OH): Penton Custom Media; 2006.

29. Medical Reserve Corps. 2016. Available at: www.medicalreservecorps.gov. Accessed March 8, 2016.

30. Centers for Disease Control and Prevention. Public health preparedness capabilities: National standards for state and local planning. Washington, DC: US Department of Health and Human Services; 2011.

31. Merchant RM, Leigh JE, Lurie N. Editorial: health care volunteers and disaster response — first, be prepared. N Engl J Med 2010;362:872–3.

32. American Red Cross. The future of American Red Cross nursing: a blueprint for action. Washington, DC: National Nursing Committee; 2012. Available at: www.redcross.org/images/MEDIA_CustomProductCatalog/m12940094_Blueprint_for_Nursing_9_2012.pdf. Accessed October, 2015.

33. Institute of Medicine. The future of nursing: leading change, advancing health. 2010. Available at: https://iom.nationalacademies.org/Reports/2010/The-Future-of-Nursing-Leading-Change-Advancing-Health.aspx. Accessed November 14, 2015.

Hospital Decontamination
What Nurses Need to Know

Brent Cox, DM, CHEP

KEYWORDS

- Hospital decontamination • Hazardous materials • Contamination
- Victim decontamination • Medical decontamination • Chemical removal

KEY POINTS

- Hospital decontamination is the removal of contaminants from a victim on arrival at the hospital.
- First receivers are caregivers or emergency personnel receiving patients for care.
- First responders are emergency personnel or caregivers going to the disaster scene or emergency area.

According to the Hazmat Intelligence Portal,[1] there were more than 15,778 hazardous material incidents with 11 deaths and 142 injuries reported by the US Department of Transportation, Pipeline and Hazardous Material Safety Administration, and the Office of Hazardous Material Safety during 2015. No mandate to track and/or report hospital decontamination responses exists; therefore, the likelihood of a greater number of hazardous material events occurring but not being reported is great. Decontamination procedures for mass casualty exposure events have traditionally focused on response at the scene versus hospital decontamination procedures and capabilities.[2] A medical center's ability to decontaminate and treat a mass influx of contaminated patients is a time-consuming and resource-exhausting task.

Times of disaster prove to be challenging for medical providers because they are looked on, by many, as the foundation of community response and recovery. Health care personnel are expected to be prepared and capable of handling any and all medical issues no matter how complex the scenario. The potential for chemical, biological, and nuclear weapons being used against the United States has steadily increased since the attacks of 9/11 and present the country with a profound threat. Although limited, research on hospital decontamination suggests concerns with hospital capabilities to adequately and safely conduct patient decontamination during incidents

Conflicts of Interest: The author has no commercial or financial conflict of interests to disclose. There is no funding source for this research.

Regional Center for Disaster Preparedness Education, College of Nursing and Health Professions, Arkansas State University, 105 North Caraway, PO Box 910, State University, Jonesboro, AR 72467, USA

E-mail address: brentcox@astate.edu

involving chemical contaminants. This article is grounded in a comprehensive literature review as well as the author's conduct of preparedness gap analysis for more than 45 hospitals and his research on hospital decontamination. The current state of medical decontamination capabilities, including a comprehensive review of literature, is elucidated and progresses to a discussion of first receiver implications for contaminated patients. In addition, suggested best practices, grounded in the evidence, are presented.

CURRENT STATE OF MEDICAL DECONTAMINATION

Current literature regarding patient care at hazardous substance incidents primarily focuses on responders who are first on the scene of the incident rather than health care professionals who provide care for the victims at hospitals. Literature available on the subject of decontamination is scarce and primarily comes from after-action reviews, agency protocols, and government standards. Most decontamination-related research and literature is derived from the first responder perspective versus that of the first receiver. Although existing literature seems to be outdated, recent evaluations of hospital preparedness support that the literature is still valid and circumstances have not improved.

Decontamination at the hospital is focused on removing all contaminants that could potentially cause secondary contamination to unprotected health care providers treating victims, current patients, and visitors.[2,3] Even after decontamination at the scene, contaminants may remain on patients' clothing or their persons.[2] When these patients then present to the hospital, medical personnel tending to them are at great risk for secondary contamination.[4] Any and all victims of an incident involving hazardous materials should be considered contaminated until health care professionals ensure that contaminants have been completely removed, regardless of on-site decontamination measures.[5] Providers should expect to receive a large number of contaminated victims, many of whom will make their way to the hospital on their own.[4–6] It is expected that up to 80% of victims in a mass casualty incident, involving contaminants or otherwise, will self-report to a medical facility.[7] In cases in which victims self-transport, hospital personnel are required to act quickly and often have little to no notice.[8]

Hospital personnel have the perception that assistance from local first responders, such as the fire department or specialized hazardous materials teams, will provide assistance with decontamination procedures and contaminant identification. This perception is a recipe for disaster. Niska[9] showed that more than 58% of medical centers intended to contact a hazardous material team for assistance during hazardous material events; however, only 44% of those medical centers conducted any form of training with hazardous material teams. Help at the hospital from responders should not be expected because responders will be deployed to the scene of the incident and not capable of sending manpower and resources elsewhere,[5] especially in rural areas where the number of first responders is limited and often depends on volunteers versus professional responders.

Kenar and Karaynlanoglu[3] suggest that the transfer of contaminated victims directly from the incident site to the hospital for treatment is a serious mistake. They reiterate that patients are generally poorly decontaminated at the scene, which creates a great potential for secondary contamination to health care workers providing direct patient care with limited protection against contaminants. Health care workers must be assured that the patients are clean and safe for direct patient contact.

A critical element of hospital safety is the ability to receive and treat contaminated or assumed contaminated victims.[2,10] Untrained and ill-prepared staff attempting to receive contaminated victims places the victims, hospital, current patients, and employees in grave danger.[10] According to Debacker,[5] the medical community has little experience with chemical agents. In order to respond accurately and effectively to a mass casualty event involving contaminated victims, specific preparedness efforts must be undertaken. The lack of these efforts, and specific resources, jeopardizes the health care facility and workers as well as the hospital's capability to respond.[11]

A case study by Hood and colleagues[2] determined that urban hospitals are minimally capable of handling contaminated patients. Therefore, the exposure rate to hospital personnel is high. Crane and colleagues[12] assessed the state of Florida's community health care providers' ability and willingness to respond to chemical or biological attacks and found that only 32.5% of Florida's health care providers have the minimal level of competency and willingness to respond. Their study further revealed that activation of the state's emergency plan would require more than 97% of the licensed health care providers to respond.[12] Despite great funding and preparation measures, hospitals remain poorly prepared for a mass influx of patients, especially if the victims are exposed to a contaminant.[13] Bennett[13] revealed that hospitals have a lack of knowledge, resources, and plans to handle small-scale incidents involving hazardous materials; therefore, a mass influx of contaminated patients will prove to be overwhelming and unmanageable. Based on existing literature and a May 2001 report produced by the American Public Health Association, less than 20% of medical facilities are prepared for victims of a chemical or biological attack.[14] George and colleagues[15] reported that, of UK emergency facilities, 90% are incapable of managing a chemical incident. Of the facilities that are capable of handling contaminated victims, most can only decontaminate 1 victim at a time using a fixed facility attached to the emergency department (ED).[5,14] Debacker[5] reported that hospital decontamination is an immense task that requires a great deal of resources, including equipment and personnel.[5] Urban hospitals tend to be better prepared for contaminated patients than rural hospitals, raising a great concern for the exposure risk in rural hospitals receiving contaminated victims.[2] It is acknowledged that, in order for response to a chemical incident to be effective, emergency preparedness must begin at the local level.[5]

IMPLICATIONS FOR FIRST RECEIVERS

A mass influx of patients presenting at the medical center produces grave concerns and challenges that must be addressed, planned for, rehearsed, and tested. Adding in a hazardous substance to the already complex issues presented by a mass casualty event not only increases the need for supplies, personnel, and assistance but adds a complexity of unknown factors as well as great safety concerns for all involved.[10]

After drills, trainings, or actual events, one of the major issues discussed in after-action reports is communication. Communication seems to be a never-ending issue and presents no less challenge during contaminated mass casualty events than any other event. Communication about the knowledge, possibility, or expectation of a hazardous substance must be relayed as soon as suspected and/or known in order to provide medical center personnel with time to prepare for the patients who will self-transport as well as be professionally transported to their facility.[7,8] This task is not easy to accomplish, because it requires collaboration and dependence on the dispatch center receiving the initial call as well as the first responders making initial assessment on arrival. Chaotic scenes such as those involving unknown hazardous substances leave little time for processing and reporting what is happening and what is to be suspected.

Once communication has been received, or patients unexpectedly begin to arrive contaminated, the hospital staff must quickly determine how to protect the facility, personnel, visitors, and current patients from cross-contamination.[2,4,5] If contaminated victims make entry into the facility before they have been decontaminated, the problem increases and the resources available diminish. Unwanted entry quickly leads to the loss of use for key areas, injury to needed personnel, as well as additional victims. Locking down the facility must occur as soon as possible; however, this is no simple endeavor. Hospitals have numerous entry points as well as emergency exits that can easily be opened by visitors, patients, or staff either accidentally or purposefully. In order to properly secure the facility and ensure that unwanted entry is not made, personnel need to be reassigned job duties in order to confirm and ensure that only 1 access point is available and that all contaminated victims are kept separate from noncontaminated victims and properly decontaminated before entry and treatment.

Caring for a mass influx of patients who are contaminated requires a robust workforce of nurses and trained personnel.[12,16] McHugh[16] explains that staffing and supporting systems are weak links within the preparedness arena. Other studies show that less than 20% of hospitals attain the knowledge and ability to decontaminate more than 1 victim at a time.[5,13–15] Staffing and maintaining a well-diversified and trained decontamination team prepared to handle a small event or a large-scale disaster involving contaminants is problematic. Employee turnover, position advancement, physical ability, and burnout are all key issues that affect the formation and sustainability of such teams. Administrators, and/or those charged with the preparedness of medical centers, should carefully consider and evaluate how they select team members and from what departments they recruit. Many facilities begin recruiting within the ED, because this is the primary impact area. By recruiting primarily from the ED, the facility is setting itself up for a snowball effect of backfilling. By pulling emergency nurses to do decontamination, nurses from elsewhere in the facility have to be pulled to staff the ED. By training a few key emergency nurses per shift to work and manage the decontamination line and pull the rest of the team members from other areas, the ED can maintain its core team to handle the medical needs of those entering the facility. Staffing a decontamination line does not have to be accomplished solely by nursing. Certified nursing assistants, facilities management personnel, occupational therapist, clinical laboratory staff, radiology technicians, home health staff, maintenance personnel, business personnel, and food services personnel are all excellent decontamination team staffing considerations (**Box 1**).

Hand in hand with staffing is the challenge of earning trust and gaining confidence for those willing to participate in the decontamination team process and become part of the team. Studies have shown that part of the reason for hospitals being unprepared is the lack of training and protocols provided to the team members.[5,12] Team training once a year, using mannequins and/or other simulated scenarios, does not provide sustainable and consistent confidence in donning and doffing the personal protective equipment, proper clothing and personal belongings removal, cleaning procedures, and/or monitoring techniques. These skills are not natural and therefore must be developed and practiced on a regular and routine training schedule in order to ensure that all members of the team are proficient and work as one.[17] Well-written, understood, and implemented processes and procedures not only assist in guiding the team members decisions but give them a foundation to build on as well as ensure they have done all that was expected and stayed within the rules, regulations, and

> **Box 1**
> **Key issues of decontamination team sustainability**
>
> - Selection of team members
> - Training
> - Protocols
> - Employee turnover
> - Position advancement
> - Physical ability
> - Burnout
> - Communication
> - Maintenance and storage of equipment
> - Decontamination location/space
> - Funding

guidelines set forth by the organization and the regulatory authorities. The lack of training and comprehensive protocols creates a mindset of not being important and/or supported and therefore leads to an untrained and ill-prepared team, if the team can sustain at all.

Along with a robust force of staff, decontamination equipment is another immense challenge for medical centers. The fight for space is a common issue and any unused area or co-usable space is quickly commandeered. This problem applies to fixed decontamination rooms as well as well-organized equipment storage areas. Fixed decontamination rooms, as well as mobile decontamination stations, must be quickly accessible and usable at a moment's notice. Many hospitals have grown accustomed to using the decontamination room as a storage area, making it time consuming to use and inaccessible to test and maintain.[18] Suits, powered air-purified respirators , batteries, brushes, soap, conveyers, mobile tents, and all the other needed supplies often get placed on the back shelves where they are difficult to get to in emergencies and easily overlooked or forgotten during safety rounds. If the needed supplies are not placed at the back of the closet they are often separated and stored in numerous locations throughout the facility, once again being difficult to locate and obtain in emergency situations. Not only is storage of the equipment an issue but maintenance of the equipment is a major obstacle as well. Decontamination equipment must be stored in the proper climate and items such as batteries must be charged, rotated, and tested on a routine basis. Hospitals were originally able to purchase and acquire needed decontamination equipment through Homeland Security funding and Hospital Preparedness grants. Although this initial investment and push increased hospital capabilities greatly, replenishing supplies such as the suits and filters was often overlooked and not budgeted, leaving facilities without new and ready suits and with expired filter cartridges.

Debacker[5] showed that 78% of hospitals acknowledge additional readiness activities that should be undertaken but are not, because of the deficiency in funding. The lack of funding allocation is thought to be caused in part by the low probability of such an event occurring at any given location. Laughrun[19] noted that administrative support for emergency planning, training, and resources was a key to success in preparing medical centers for such emergencies. Without administrative buy-in, preparedness activities such as decontamination capabilities will not be enhanced and improved on. Administration has to acknowledge the need and importance of proper equipment, training, and protocols to ensure that, when such an event occurs, the safety of the staff members, patients, and visitors to the facility are protected and treated to the best of the medical center's ability. Although the training and equipment are expensive, the cost/benefit analysis leans in favor of preparedness versus last minute response.

BEST PRACTICES

With all the immense challenges facing medical centers and health care providers, it is easy to become overwhelmed and question where to start and how to begin preparing for such an extensive and complex task. Although caring for contaminated victims may seem to be an impossible and/or an exhaustive task, there are many evidence-based steps and processes that can be taken. Following these best practices assists in ensuring the implementation of a comprehensive and well-prepared plan, policies, procedures, as well as a trained and confident decontamination team equipped to handle the challenges that will present.

When considering ways to strengthen a medical center's capabilities and reduce an identified gap, a key component to success is to establish and ensure upper administration buy-in and complete support.[13,16,19] This component alone can be a difficult challenge to overcome. Administration is focused on the bottom line and ensuring that financial support is making the greatest impact for the dollar. Key administrators should be kept enlightened on the increasing number of contaminated victims and potential for such an event to occur. At the same time, administrators should understand that the number of hospital decontamination incidents is not well reported and therefore most likely represent a very small portion of actual contaminated incidents. Administrators should be brought in on the beginning stages of the development or restructuring process in order to gain a complete understanding of the need and potential impact on the facility, staff, patients, visitors, and community as a whole.

Policy development is another key element of successful decontamination teams. A diverse and educated team that understands the inner workings of the facility, as well as the community needs and capabilities, should develop the policy and procedure document. The policy team should include a representative from all key departments within the medical center to ensure that an action or process does not hinder or jeopardize the processes required or expected within other key departments. The policy committee should attempt to be all-inclusive and consider all possible scenarios. Policy and procedure documents should include topics such as[20–25]:

- The decision to decontaminate
- Activation
- Outside resource request
- Preparation procedure and administrative process
- Team qualifications, training, and requirements
- Equipment maintenance program
- Crowd control
- Decontamination operation procedures
- Patient care procedures
- Internal contamination management
- Special population considerations
- Contaminated dead
- Personal belongings/evidence collection
- Technical decontamination
- Radioactive incidents

- Environmental concerns
- Restocking
- Staff debriefing

Notification and communication is a key piece to successfully completing this complex puzzle of preparedness. Collaboration and teamwork with all involved in hazardous substance incidents is essential. Medical center personnel should be discussing, training with, and drilling all aspects of the notification, response, and recovery cycles with all participants to ensure that the entire picture is understood and each organization's roles and needs are addressed. In order to decrease the gap in communication, especially considering early notification of possible contamination, the process must be openly examined and put into all agencies' policies and procedures, then practiced and tested in high-stress reenactments to ensure that the process works and is used.[19]

Throughout the medical center, equipment is strategically analyzed, monitored, and maintained. Decontamination equipment should be no different than a patient's ventilator or any other lifesaving tool that clinicians use. An all-inclusive maintenance and evaluation program should be established and routinely updated.[23] The maintenance program should include physical inspection of all equipment, ensuring that all components are properly labeled and located in their designated places. The inspection process should also include all components to ensure that no damage has occurred as well as testing all motorized or working parts to ensure proper function. Batteries should be routinely rotated on and off chargers and used to ensure proper function. Water, heaters, pumps, hoses, sprayers, and all other equipment should be physically tested and not just assumed to function properly.[23]

Team development should be considered a priority and given special attention. Those in administration should think outside the box when recruiting for decontamination teams and expand their scope beyond the ED and certified nurses. Pay increases and special bonuses may be beyond an organization's ability; however, other forms of recognition and special benefits can show value and appreciation to the employees who accept assignment to a decontamination team. Ideas for decontamination members include special parking privileges, unique identification cards, extended breaks, or other privileged perks. Potential departments from which to recruit decontamination team members include:

- Environmental services
- Maintenance
- Physical therapy
- Occupational therapy
- Laboratory
- Pharmacy
- Business office
- Education
- Wellness center
- Home health
- Obstetrics/gynecology
- Information technology
- Medical records

Training should be a priority for anyone involved with the decontamination process at any level. Training has to be constantly evolving and continuous. When designing and considering who to train and what training should be provided, tunnel vision should be avoided. Training is not specific to decontamination team members but must be outreaching to all arms of the organization. It is vital for front desk clerks, security personnel, and any employee who may come into contact with presenting victims to understand how to recognize a possible contamination and what to do if contamination is expected.[23,24,26] Team members should be training individually and as a team. Training should include didactic content in which policies, procedures, best practices, and recent research is covered, as well as hands-on practical application. Hands-on training should be as realistic as possible and advance into high-stress practical situations. Training coordinators should be diligent in ensuring that training is conducted in the same manner in which real-life situations will be handled.

Understanding the proper process and procedures to implement and follow during contaminated events and using the same systematic approach each time builds team confidence and functionality. Recommended and evidence-based procedures for the hospital decontamination process include[20–25]:

- Recognition of need for decontamination.
- If more than 1 victim, implement security measures to secure facility.
- Activate decontamination team and support staff.
- Decontamination team dons personal protective equipment.
- Support staff prepares decontamination corridor, zones, and supplies.
- Establish triage area and display predetermined instructional script for victims.
- Once the triage team and decontamination team are prepared, begin processing patients.
- Triage patients based on a combination of injury and contaminant severity.
- Only perform lifesaving care during triage and decontamination process.
- Move patients to appropriate area, such as ambulatory or nonambulatory line.
- Using a premade or purchased kit, identify the patient by using a barcode, bracelet, numbering system, or other form of identification.
- Remove clothing by carefully cutting in a top-down fashion, making smooth cuts and not ripping (**Fig. 1**).
- Clothing should be removed after cutting. Roll the material inside out and off the patient. Make sure the hazardous substance is contained inside the material (**Fig. 2**).

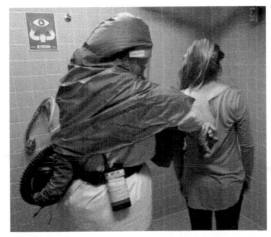

Fig. 1. Cut out. (*Courtesy of* Arkansas State University, Regional Center for Disaster Preparedness Education; with permission.)

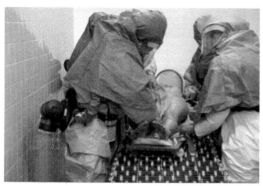

Fig. 2. Clothing removal. (*Courtesy of* Arkansas State University, Regional Center for Disaster Preparedness Education; with permission.)

- The patient should then be rolled from left to right in order to remove the clothing completely from the victim.
- Clothing should be bagged, tagged, and stored in a hazardous material container and safeguarded as possible evidence.
- Any and all jewelry, including piercings, rings, watches, necklaces, and hair pieces, that can safely be removed should be removed and placed into a property bagged and tagged as to who it belongs to (**Fig. 3**). The personal items should then be placed in a hazardous material storage bin specifically designated for personal belongings.
- Once all clothing and personal belongings have been removed, the victim should be thoroughly rinsed from head to toe, taking precautions to protect the respiratory system (**Fig. 4**).
- Thorough washing should begin using soap, water, and brushes (**Fig. 5**).
- One soap bucket and brush should be designated for the head. Each team member should have a brush and access to a bucket of soapy water.
- The team member responsible for the head uses copious amounts of water and soap to thoroughly wash the hair, face, and neck. Brush strokes should pull the contaminant away from the victim, working in a downward motion from the center of the body to the outside. The team member with responsibility for the head works from the top of the head to the patient's collar bone.

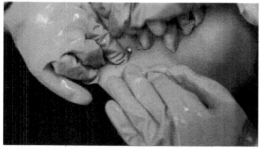

Fig. 3. Object removal. (*Courtesy of* Arkansas State University, Regional Center for Disaster Preparedness Education; with permission.)

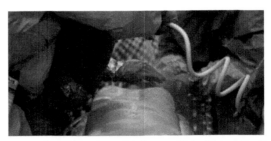

Fig. 4. Respiratory protection. (*Courtesy of* Arkansas State University, Regional Center for Disaster Preparedness Education; with permission.)

- With 2 team members on each side of the victim, the upper body members work from the chin to the waistline and from the center of the body outward. The team members with responsibility for the lower half of the body work from the navel to the toes. After each brush stroke the brush should be dipped and rinsed in soapy water.
- Once the front portion of the patient has been completely and thoroughly scrubbed, the team rolls the patient from left to right, washing the back of the patient and ensuring that all portions of the body have been scrubbed.
- Team members' hands should be cleaned each time they touch the patient. If the patient is on a spine board, the board must be cleaned before the patient is rolled back onto the surface.
- Once the patient has been washed and is deemed to be clean, the patient should be placed on a clean spine board, covered, and transported into the medical center for treatment.

Preparing for hospital decontamination is an ongoing and never-ending cycle that must be continuously evaluated and trained for. Ongoing hazard vulnerability analysis (HVA), including common contaminants in the geographic region, should be routinely conducted both for the facility as well as the community.[23,26] The HVA should guide decontamination preparedness activities. After any and all real-life scenarios or training exercises, an after-action review should be conducted and used to guide future education and training.[19]

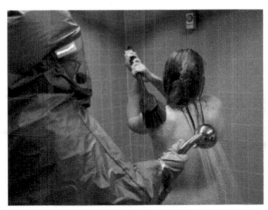

Fig. 5. Thorough cleanse. (*Courtesy of* Arkansas State University, Regional Center for Disaster Preparedness Education; with permission.)

SUMMARY

An influx of mass-casualty contaminated victims presenting at the hospital at a moment's notice is an ever-increasing threat to medical centers and the health care personnel who provide care and support. Although this is a complex and difficult task, by preplanning and implementing strategic strategies, policies, procedures, education, and training, medical centers can strengthen their capabilities and lessen the current gap in hospital decontamination capabilities.

REFERENCES

1. US Department of Transportation. 2016 Pipeline and hazardous materials safety. Available at: https://portal.phmsa.dot.gov. Accessed May 10, 2016.
2. Hood J, Fernandes-Flack J, Larranaga MD. Effectiveness of hospital-based decontamination during a simulated mass casualty exposure. J Occup Environ Hyg 2011;8:D131–8.
3. Kenar JL, Karayilanoglu T. A Turkish Medical Rescue Team against nuclear, biological, and chemical weapons. Mil Med 2004;169(2):94–6.
4. Horton DK, Burgess P, Rossiter S, et al. Secondary contamination of emergency department personnel from o-chlorobenzylidene malononitrile exposure, 2002. Ann Emerg Med 2005;45(6):655–8.
5. Debacker M. Hospital preparedness for incidents with chemical agents. Int J Disast Med 2003;1:42–50.
6. Williams G, Williams E. A nursing guide to surviving a radiological dispersal device. Br J Nurs 2010;19(1):24–7.
7. Moffett PM, Baker BL, Kang CS, et al. Evaluation of time required for water-only decontamination of an oil-based agent. Mil Med 2010;175(3):185–7.
8. Al-Damouk M, Bleetman A. Impact of the department of health initiative to equip and train acute trusts to manage chemically contaminated casualties. Emerg Med J 2005;22:347–50.
9. Niska RW. Hospital collaboration with public safety organizations on bioterrorism response. Prehosp Emerg Care 2008;12:12–7.
10. Edwards D, Williams L, Beatty J, et al. First-receiver hospital decontamination; an 8-step approach to a progressive and practical program. J Nurs Adm 2007;37(3): 122–30.
11. Remmen JV. Hospital treatment capacity for casualties exposed to irritant gases in the Netherlands. Int J Disast Med 2005;1(4):32–6.
12. Crane JS, McCluskey JD, Johnson GT, et al. Assessment of community healthcare providers ability and willingness to respond to emergencies resulting from bioterrorist attacks. J Emerg Trauma Shock 2010;3(1):13–20.
13. Bennett RL. Chemical or biological terrorist attacks: an analysis of the preparedness of hospitals for managing victims affected by chemical or biological weapons of mass destruction. Int J Environ Res Public Health 2006;3(1):67–75.
14. Gluckman WA, Rosania A, McDonald W. An approach to hospital decontamination team development at a university hospital. Int J Disast Med 2004;2:48–51.
15. George G, Ramsay K, Rochester M, et al. Facilities for chemical decontamination in accident and emergency departments in the United Kingdom. Emerg Med J 2002;19:453–7.
16. McHugh MD. Hospital nurse staffing and public health emergency preparedness: implications for policy. Public Health Nurs 2010;27(5):442–9.
17. Federal Emergency Management Agency. Framework for healthcare emergency management. Center for Domestic Preparedness.

18. Bendele K. Arkansas state gap analysis. Little Rock (AR): Arkansas Department of Health; 2013.
19. Laughrun GM. Preparing your hospital to respond to a terrorist attack. Am J Health Syst Pharm 2002;59:1329–30.
20. Continuum Health Partners. Hospital decontamination of exposed casualties policy and procedure. New York: Assistant Secretary for Preparedness & Response, US Government; 2006.
21. Victorian Government Initiative. Decontamination guidance for hospitals. Melbourne (Australia): Victoria Department of Human Services; 2007.
22. Starling C. Recommendations for hospitals: chemical decontamination, staff protection, chemical decontamination equipment and medication list and evidence collection. Rancho Cordova (CA): Emergency Medical Services Authority; 2003.
23. OSHA. 2005 OSHA best practices for hospital-based first receivers of victims from mass casualty incidents involving the release of hazardous substances. Available at: https://www.osha.gov/dts/osta/bestpractices/html/hospital_firstreceivers. html. Accessed May 12, 2016.
24. Georgia Hospital. Decontamination program guidance. Atlanta (GA): Georgia Hospital; 2014.
25. Harvard School of Public Health. Hospital decontamination self-assessment tool. Cambridge (MA): Emergency Preparedness and Response Exercise Program; 2014.
26. Powers R. Organization of a hospital-based victim decontamination plan using the incident command structure. Disaster Manag Response 2007;5(4):119–23.

Radiation, Fear, and Common Sense Adaptations in Patient Care

Robert C. Beauchamp, BSN, RN, CEN, EMT-P

KEYWORDS

- Radiation • Ionizing radiation • Contamination • Exposure • Fear • Safety
- Adaptations in nursing care

KEY POINTS

- Lack of understanding of the nature of ionizing radiation has resulted in fear among health care providers regarding the care of patients contaminated with radioactive material.
- Such fear and misunderstanding can lead to unnecessary compromises in patient care.
- Caregiver and patient safety is ensured by an understanding of the basic science of radiation and common sense alterations in normal nursing technique.

FEAR AND ALL HAZARDS

Appropriate fear may limit the spread of a deadly disease.[1] The outbreaks of the Ebola virus have rightly rekindled fears of biological agents. CNN quoted the World Health Organization as saying that 416 medical caregivers had contracted the disease with 233 dying.[2] Fear of contracting Ebola by cross contamination is well founded. In 1995, the sarin nerve agent attack in Tokyo generated widespread fear about the dangers of chemical terrorism. This event became a watershed for warnings about imminent attacks and the need for mass casualty chemical training.[3] The need to be prepared for "all hazards" has led many hospitals to adopt "Level A" precautions for all chemical, biological, or radiation events.[3]

However, this level of fear is not appropriate in the case of a properly managed radiation event. The most likely accident results from a mishandled radiation source or an injury occurring in a contaminated work area.[4] For example, in 1987, an abandoned radioactive medical source was broken open by individuals in search of valuable scrap material in Goiania, Brazil. As a result, 249 people were contaminated with Cesium137. More than 100 were internally contaminated and 20 people had to be

Disclosure: None.
Radiation Emergency Assistance Center/Training Site (REAC/TS), Oak Ridge Associated Universities, PO Box 117, MS 39, Oak Ridge, TN 37831, USA
E-mail address: Robert.Beauchamp@orau.org

hospitalized to treat the effects of high radiation exposure. Four of these people died.[5] The medical staff and public responses were marked by fear and panic. Some patients were isolated in a ward for 24 hours without food and water. One patient was left overnight in an ambulance outside the hospital.[6] A team of physicians from the National Nuclear Energy Commission arrived and began working with little support from the health care community. Local training was provided and some staff did volunteer for treatment team duties. Even so, the fear of radiation was so profound that many staff members still refused and even called the volunteers "suicidal."[7]

WHAT IS RADIATION?

Radiation is energy transmitted through a medium. Examples are sound, light, radio waves, and micro waves. These are not ionizing radiations.

Ionizing radiation has enough energy to strip electrons from the outer shells of atoms, thus creating an ion and making the atom more chemically reactive with its neighbors. These free radicals may result in indirect damage to living tissue.[8] In some instances, radiation may cause a break in the DNA strand of a living cell. This direct damage may make it impossible for the cell to multiply, thus causing cell death. It is possible that DNA damage may cause a mutation that is passed on to successive generations, thus increasing the chances of cancer at some future point.[8] It should be noted that our bodies are well adapted to repairing radiation damage. We live in a universe in which radiation is everywhere. It is in the dirt, in food, in air, and throughout the universe as cosmic rays.[9] The point of radiation safety is to prevent exposure to an amount of radiation that would overwhelm our natural repair mechanisms.

An element is determined by the number of protons in the nucleus. If the ratio of neutrons to protons is not stable the atom will release radiation as it decays to a stable state.[8] For example, stable Iodine (I-127) has 53 protons and 74 neutrons. But Iodine131 has 4 more neutrons, is unstable and emits radiation. Radioactive Iodine is still chemically the same as stable Iodine. The chemical nature of any material is unaffected by the fact that it is radioactive.

AN ATOM MAY DECAY IN DIFFERENT WAYS

Alpha radiation is the emission of an alpha particle from the nucleus. An alpha particle consists of 2 protons and 2 neutrons. This strong 2^+ charge means alpha radiation gives up its energy quickly. It can only travel centimeters in air and is easily shielded, even by a piece of paper.[10] Alpha radiation cannot penetrate intact skin and is not an external threat. But if an alpha-emitting material were internalized it would be in immediate contact with living cells and would be a threat. A primary goal is to prevent or minimize internalization. Examples of alpha-emitting materials are Plutonium 238, Americium 241, and Polonium 210.[11,12]

Beta radiation is the emission of a beta particle (electron) from the nucleus of the atom. Beta radiation is more penetrating than alpha radiation, and can travel up to a meter in air or cause radiation damage to the skin. It cannot penetrate internal organs or bone marrow. Eyeglasses and heavier clothing are sufficient shielding for most beta radiation. An example of a beta-emitting material is Strontium 90.[11,12]

Gamma radiation is not a subatomic particle but pure energy (measured as "photons"). It is less ionizing and, therefore, more penetrating than alpha or beta radiation. Gamma radiation travels many meters in air and requires feet of concrete and inches of lead for shielding. This makes it an external threat in sufficient doses. Gamma rays have a wide variety of energies that are specific to the given isotope, its own finger print. An unknown gamma emitter can be identified by using a gamma spectrometer.

Examples of gamma emitters are Iridium 192 and Cobalt 60.[11,12] **Fig. 1** illustrates the penetrating nature of alpha, beta, gamma and neutron radiation.

X-rays may be viewed as similar to gamma radiation. The primary difference is that X-rays are machine generated. X-rays are emitted only when the X-ray machine is energized.[12]

Finally, in some special cases, a radioactive material may decay by ejecting a neutron. However, the chances of neutron radiation becoming an issue for the basic nursing care of a contaminated patient are remote and is not discussed in this article.

It should be noted that the preceding discussion of ionizing radiation has been intentionally kept at a basic conceptual level. Some texts for those who would study further are *Basic Radiation Technology* by Daniel Golnick[13] and *Radiation Threats and Your Safety* by Arman Ansari.[12]

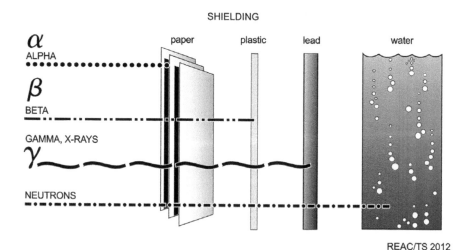

REAC/TS 2012

Fig. 1. Penetrating characteristics.

EXPOSURE VERSUS CONTAMINATION

Simply stated, exposure is being in the presence of ionizing radiation. One is exposed to radiation when receiving a radiograph or when near radioactive material. Contamination is the result of getting radioactive material on or in your person. If you are near a radioactive material and you leave the area, you are no longer being exposed. This may sound very simple, but it is an important concept that many caregivers do not appreciate and bears repeating. Exposure is being in the presence of radioactivity and contamination is getting a radioactive material on or in your person.[14]

DETECTION

The ionization of atoms is the freeing of electrons from their orbital shells, which is an electrical event. Thus, detecting the presence of radiation is a simple matter. There are many types of detection devices that can demonstrate the presence of above-normal radiation levels. One of the earliest is a standard Geiger counter (GM) meter, pictured in **Fig. 2**. They are manufactured by a number of different companies in varying degrees of complexity.

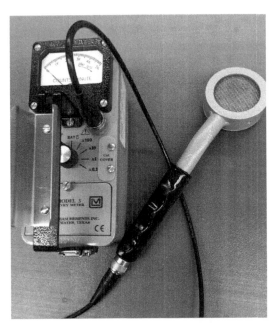

Fig. 2. Standard Geiger counter (GM) meter.

A survey meter is used to quickly determine the presence of radioactive contamination and, in the hands of an experienced user, characterize the material as an alpha, beta, or gamma emitter. Every emergency department (ED) should have at least 1 survey meter, and staff should be properly trained in its use.

SAFETY

Basic radiation safety guidelines are simple. Most of us have heard of "time, distance, and shielding." To this concept, we also add the concept of quantity. Limit time in a radiation area to necessary duties and increase your distance from a radiation source. The intensity of radioactivity is inversely proportional to the square of the distance from the source. If you double your distance away from a source you are receiving 4 times less radiation dose. If you double the distance back again, you are 16 times safer and so on. If you are not involved in the immediate care of a contaminated patient, take a step or 2 back.

Quantity is also an important concept. When a patient presents with radioactive material on his or her clothing, bagging the clothing and removing it from the area reduces the radiation dose for everyone.

Shielding is not practical in the patient treatment scenario. For instance, the lead vests used in the radiology department are designed to protect from lower-energy X-rays. Gamma radiation is typically more energetic and the vests will not be an effective shield. In addition, they are tiresome to wear for extended periods of time.

It is difficult to imagine a scenario in which a patient has so much radioactive material on their person that he or she represents a serious threat to caregivers who exercise the safety principles mentioned previously. Even at Chernobyl, as noted by the Department of Homeland Security Working Group on Radiological Dispersal Device Preparedness.

"Based on the Chernobyl experience, once a person has been removed from the radiation area, it is very unlikely that particulate radioactivity or radioactive fallout will result in a significant hazard to attendants who are wearing protective garb. Doses received by Chernobyl attendants were in the range of 10 mSv (0.01 Gy). The most effective quick method of reducing external contamination and decreasing attendant exposure is removal of the external clothing. This should be done as soon as practical. The clothing should be bagged and tagged."[15]

The international units of 1 Gy or 1 Sievert equal 100 rad or 100 rem in US units. These victims were heavily contaminated, yet the dose to medical attendants was very low at 0.01 Gy or 1 rad. This is one-fifth of the 5-rad (0.05 Gy) regulatory dose allowed for a US radiation worker every year![16] Significant contamination events can be handled safely with time, distance, and reducing quantity by bagging and removing contaminated material to a secured area.

PUTTING IT ALL TOGETHER

Using these principles and the experience gained from actual responses over the past 42 years, the Radiation Emergency Assistance Center Training Site (REAC/TS) (**Box 1**) has designed the patient flow chart shown in **Fig. 3**. It is not a step-by-step set of definitive regulations but a logical flow of patient care based on science and historical events. It is downloadable at https://orise.orau.gov/files/reacts/radiation-patient-treatment-algorithm.pdf. Let's apply it to actual patient scenarios.

SCENARIO 1

As mentioned earlier, a common accident scenario involves sealed sources. Pipe welds, can be examined by using a radioactive source inside the pipe and wrapping X-ray film around the outside.[17] Highly radioactive sources can be used to sterilize food or medical supplies.[18] These sources can be very dangerous and should be stored in a "safe" position in a shielded case or lowered into a water-filled pool.

A worker at a food sterilization facility has entered the working area to unstick a belt that moves products around a radiation source. Somehow the source is in the raised position and the safety alarms failed to sound. While up on a ladder the worker realizes the situation and in his panic to leave, falls and possibly breaks his ankle. He crawls from the area and calls for help. Coworkers make sure the source is lowered into the shielding and call for an ambulance (loosely based on an actual accident in Belarus).[19] The patient is in transit with his vital signs stable and his ankle splinted. The paramedics report that the patient has vomited while en route (approximately 30 to 40 minutes after leaving the radiation area). What should nursing staff do? What changes do they have to make to protect themselves from this patient?

This situation requires the caregivers to remember the difference between contamination and exposure. This patient has been exposed to a sealed source. Once the

---

Box 1
Radiation Emergency Assistance Center Training Site (REAC/TS) information

REAC/TS is an international resource in the medical management of radiation emergencies. REAC/TS provides incident response and consultation, continuing medical education and simulation exercises to countries around the globe. REAC/TS, a US Department of Energy emergency response asset, also provides assistance and expertise to federal and state agencies as well as hospitals and first responders in preparing for incidents involving human exposure to radiation.

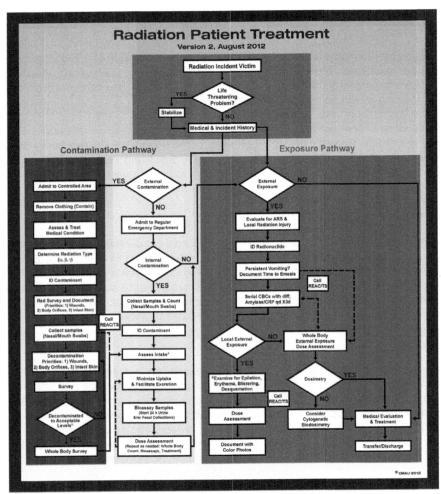

Fig. 3. Radiation patient treatment algorithm. [a] See REAC/TS pocket guide http://orise.orau. gov/reacts/resources/radiation-accident-managerment.aspx. [b] <2 to 3 times natural background or no reduction in counts, medical priorities dictate stopping decontamination, health physics consultation warranted.

patient left the area he was no longer being exposed and does not have any radioactive material on his person.

Using the treatment flow chart seen in **Fig. 3**, we use the exposure side of the chart on the right. There is no immediate life-threatening problem and we know that he is not contaminated because he was exposed to a sealed source. The ED steps are as follows: take a complete history, document time to vomiting, and draw laboratories to include a first complete blood count with total lymphocyte count. This should be repeated every 2 to 3 hours during the first 8 hours after a known exposure and every 4 to 6 hours for the next 2 days. Used together, these are the best early indicators of significant radiation exposure.[20,21] A precipitous drop in the lymphocyte count is a sensitive marker for impending acute radiation syndrome. Give symptomatic support, consider reverse isolation, admit for follow-up with Hematology and other appropriate services to deal with a possibly immune-compromised patient. No special changes in normal nursing care are necessary to treat the patient who has only been exposed to radiation.

Based on the accident description and early vomiting, our patient may have received a very high dose. A reconstruction of the event, the strength of the source, the identity of the nuclide, the patient's distance to the source, and the time exposed will be reconstructed with health physics support. The worker's dosimetry badge will be analyzed to get an actual dose reading; however, these results may not be available for hours to days in some cases.

SCENARIO 2

Your ED is informed that a workplace accident victim is en route from a radioactive waste disposal center. While welding a lid on a barrel of contaminated waste, a small explosion occurred and the material caught fire. The fire was extinguished almost immediately. The company's health physicist told emergency medical services (EMS) crew, "the patient is contaminated but not seriously and they need to get him to the hospital." Note: health physicists are specialists in radiation safety.[22] They work in industrial, medical, and many other settings. Visit The Health Physics Society Web site at http://hps.org.

EMS has reported a 48-year-old man who was doing the welding. The ambulance crew found him sitting up as he had walked away from the event approximately 20 to 30 feet to a bench. He has bruising to his left rib cage and complains of buzzing and ringing in his ears with a headache and also complains of pain on deep inspiration. He has a laceration to his left lower leg and bleeding has stopped. Heart rate 110...respiratory rate 16...blood pressure 140/88. He is awake and responsive and states he does remember the explosion and denies loss of consciousness. No care has been given beyond the wound dressing and oxygen. Their estimated time of arrival is 20 minutes.

HOW DO YOU PREPARE? IS THIS A DANGEROUS SITUATION?

Let's apply what we have learned. These people worked in close proximity to the barrel containing radioactive material and the health physicist with the patient did not exhibit any concern over high radiation dose rates. We do not suspect there is a high-level radiation source involved. Further calls for information should be made to the company for the identity and activity of the nuclide(s).

As we prepare, it may be helpful to think of what you would do if a patient was covered in smelly swamp muck from a boating accident. First, save the patient and then deal with the offensive material as soon as practical. A treatment room will be designated as our contaminated room and the patient can come in a separate entrance. If your hospital has a decontamination room, be certain that critical interventions can be performed immediately in that area. When appropriate we will decontaminate, but lifesaving always comes first![22]

In **Fig. 4**, a paper pathway from the ambulance bay to the treatment room has been placed. This may help with eventual clean-up but is not a required step. When finished, someone will still have to survey the floor clean and, unlike biological or chemical spills, any spots of radioactive contamination can usually just be wiped up. If your protocols call for paper, be sure to securely tape all the edges. Removing unnecessary equipment may reduce the time spent on clean-up efforts.

As seen in **Fig. 5**, the beds have multiple waterproof sheets. A number of trash cans with large plastic bag liners with radiation and bio-hazard warning labels should be

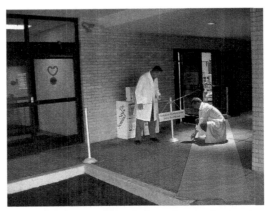

Fig. 4. Paper pathway entrance from the ambulance bay to the treatment room.

pre-positioned. The floor in the room has been covered with paper and a cart with some extra supplies has been prepared. These include extra 4 × 4 gauze sponges, adhesive drapes, extra absorbent pads, plastic sample bags, irrigation supplies, mild soap, tape, dosimeters, and a meter. This is about all that is needed to deal with a patient contaminated with radioactive material.

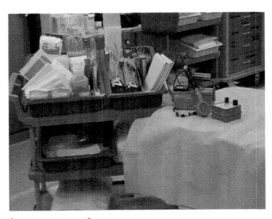

Fig. 5. Supplies and room preparation.

Is it necessary for the receiving nurses to dress in chemical protection suits with supplied air? Unless there is a chemical hazard in addition to radioactive contamination the answer would be "no." The fabric of a chemical protection suit offers no protection against gamma radiation and likely will make the responding nurse subject to heat stress.[23] Inhalation threat is determined by the chemical and physical nature of the material and the type of radiation being emitted. If internalized, alpha emitters can be 20 times more biologically damaging than gamma emitters.[8] Liquids, chunks of metal, and pebbles are not likely to become suspended in the air. If, on the other hand, the material is a fine powder, we may have more concern about airway protection. Ideally, an air sampler is running and regularly checked. However, these are not routinely available in an ED.

Remember the saying, "What goes up must come down?" A quick check can be done after the patient arrives. If there is airborne contamination, it should show on a wipe from the floor or the bottom of the caregiver's feet. If surveying these wipes is negative, there is probably very little or no radioactive material in the air. If we find contamination with these checks we should be stricter about airway precautions. From a radiation/contamination protection standpoint, an N-95 mask should be adequate airway protection. Naturally, a powered air purifying respirator (PAPR) would do the job too, but these make communication difficult and may be alarming to the patient. Remember that anyone using an N-95 or PAPR must be fit tested per the Occupational Safety and Health Administration (OSHA) guidelines. (OSHA's Respiratory Protection Standard 29 CFR 1910.134).[24] As always, follow your hospital's protocol for airway protection.

Fig. 6 shows preparation with ordinary hospital scrubs. The nurse is double-gloved with inner gloves and booties taped and wearing a surgical mask with splash shield and head cover. In most cases this would be adequate to ensure we do not get either blood or radioactive contamination on our personal clothes or splashed in the face. Fig. 7 shows another option, using paper coveralls. If you need to move quickly, a scrub gown or a plastic apron with double gloves could get you started until life-threatening problems are stabilized. As previously noted, if the contaminate is easily airborne, an N-95 would replace the surgical mask.

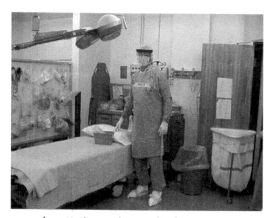

Fig. 6. Scrubs for personal protective equipment (PPE).

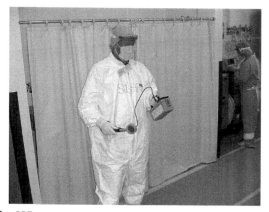

Fig. 7. Coveralls for PPE.

On patient arrival, nursing actions are prioritized using the REAC/TS algorithm as a guide (see **Fig. 3**). Life-threatening problems are stabilized as soon as they are found. This is the normal sequence in any patient survey. Critical airway, breathing, or circulation problems are fixed immediately before moving on.[25]

In **Fig. 8**, the patient has arrived wearing his work clothes. Medical caregivers assess his airway, circulation, and mental acuity. If no immediate life threats are present, for the moment the patient is stable. During the initial medical assessment, our radiation technician (or whoever is using the meter) makes a quick scan of the patient. Holding the meter 0.5 inch over the patient's clothing, the technician scans up the centerline looking for any counts above background. The bloody wound dressing also would be quickly checked. Notice that the technician stays out of the way of medical assessment of life-threatening problems. This survey is only to determine if contamination is present. A complete and detailed contamination survey will be performed only after the patient's clothing is removed. The radiation technician informs the medical team that the patient does have contamination on his clothing.

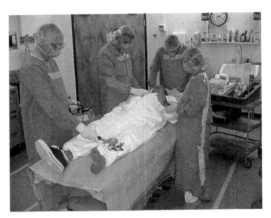

Fig. 8. First contact.

Using the treatment flow chart (see **Fig. 3**), we have decided the patient is initially stable, but he is contaminated. We work our way down both sides of the flow chart for contamination and exposure.

As we begin removing the clothing, do not forget to ask about allergies, medicines, and medical and surgical history. There is always a temptation to focus on the contamination, especially if the radiation survey meter is making noise. In **Fig. 9**, the patient's airway has been protected by putting a splash shield upside down on his face. If he were wearing an oxygen mask, then his airway would be covered. Remember, the best way to control contamination is to be careful while removing clothing. No tearing and ripping or throwing on the floor. The patient's clothes are carefully cut from head toward feet (**Fig. 10**). The clothes are rolled away from the patient to contain and trap contamination (**Fig. 11**). After touching contaminated clothes, the outer gloves are changed before touching clean skin. The patient is log rolled and the clothes are contained in the top sheet (**Fig. 12**).

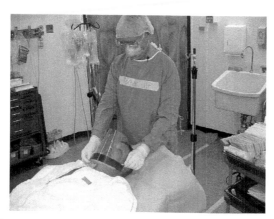

Fig. 9. Face cover.

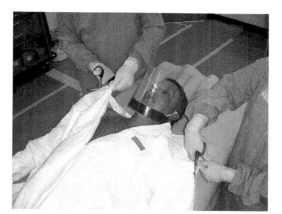

Fig. 10. Cutting clothes.

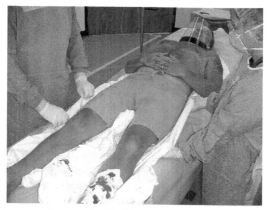

Fig. 11. Roll clothing away from patient's skin.

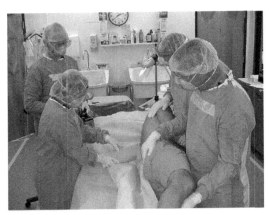

Fig. 12. Gathering contaminated clothing in top sheet.

The contaminated clothing is carefully bagged and labeled, then double-bagged as it is passed through the control line. This is an important sample, as most of the contamination will be on the patient's clothes. Bagging and removing the clothes reduces the amount of radioactive material in the room and therefore reduces the dose to everyone. This material may be sent to a gamma spectrometer for identification or held for evidence.

With the clothes removed, the patient is now held in the last log roll position on a clean sheet. The medical team performs a head-to-toe trauma survey and the radiation technician can survey the patient's back (**Fig. 13**). This survey is done quickly to look for any high contamination areas, but the radiation technician is careful to let the medical team's trauma survey have priority.

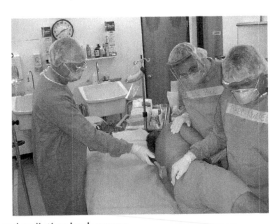

Fig. 13. Trauma and radiation back survey.

Referring again to our flow chart (see **Fig. 3**), on the exposure and contamination pathway, a number of things happen at once. The most important step after removing the clothing is the "Assess and Treat Medical Condition" directive. Now we want to obtain complete vital signs, listen to lung sounds, and examine the abdomen. Intravenous lines (IVs) should be started if needed and laboratories drawn. A priority laboratory test will be a complete blood count with differential; we will be looking for any drop in lymphocyte count over the next 24 to 48 hours. Any nausea or vomiting should be documented.

Is this material an alpha, beta, or gamma emitter? A knowledgeable radiation survey technician should be able to determine the type of radiation being emitted. Contact the work site and get more information about the nature and identity of the material in the drum.

Although the patient does not immediately appear unstable, we must not forget that the mechanism of injury was some type of explosion. There could be internal injuries. If the ED physician wants a computed tomography (CT) or other emergent study, those take priority (**Fig. 14**). Cocoon the patient in the sheet and move immediately to perform the necessary study. A call ahead to the CT or MRI will give them time to put a paper sheet on the table and don a scrub gown and gloves. Careful technique will minimize the chance of spreading contamination.

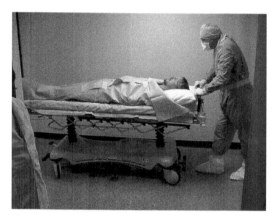

Fig. 14. Cocoon and stat transport to CT.

The explosive mechanism and contamination on clothing certainly suggests possible internal contamination. As soon as possible, the radiation technician should survey the patient's face. If there has been an inhalation, contamination will normally be evident on the face.

In **Fig. 15**, nasal swabs of each nare are taken and checked for contamination. This is not an attempt to decontaminate the nose. It is to see if there is a possible inhalation exposure. If the patient's nose needs to be cleared the patient can be encouraged to do a vigorous nose blow. Each swab should be labeled left or right, surveyed for counts per minute, individually bagged, and documented. If these samples are obtained within the first hour, they can be used to estimate the inhalation intake. Estimating possible inhalation intake depends on the nature of the material, particle size, meter efficiency, and other variable factors. See the REAC/TS Web site for further information or call for consult. The point is to remember to take the swab samples and document the counts per minute and the time.

Once the chemical safety of the material has been confirmed, there are numerous methods for inhibiting absorption and uptake in the gut that are used routinely in all EDs. Also, with internal contamination, there are medicines that can help the body excrete the material once it has been identified. For Cesium[137] we use an oral medicine called Prussian Blue or Radiogardase. For Plutonium and Americium, an IV medicine called diethylene triamine pentaacetic acid (DTPA) is used.[10] A detailed

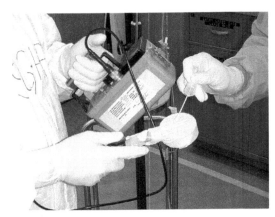

Fig. 15. Nares swab check.

discussion of internal contamination and treatment is not possible here. The point to remember is to identify the material as soon as possible. Consult with your health physics support or call REAC/TS.

After samples are secured, nursing care continues by following the "Exposure" side of the REAC/TS patient algorithm, we are approximately half way down. Our patient is awake and alert and denies any history of nausea or vomiting. He is showing no symptoms of a large external exposure and we would not expect any from our reports of the incident. We have drawn our laboratories and continue to monitor vital signs and support him per our normal routine. Information on the isotope and material in the barrel will help with care planning. Radiation workers should be wearing personal dosimeters, and should obtain a reading as soon as possible. Finally, the health physicist at the scene should be able to give us more information from his reconstruction/analysis of the accident events.

On the "Contamination" side of the REAC/TS patient algorithm, we have collected nasal swabs and sent the clothing for analysis. The radiation technician should have identified if this material is an alpha, beta, or gamma emitter. If the patient remains medically stable, move to evaluate his leg wound. The GM meter has shown counts above background over the wound dressing and if the wound itself is contaminated, it is first on the decontamination priority list.

Fig. 16 shows tongs being used to remove the dressing. Maximizing distance minimizes dose. This wound dressing is another important sample. It is bagged, checked with a meter, and **Fig. 17** shows it ready to send across the control line.

The next priority is to survey the wound and document the beginning count rate. The wound can be flushed per normal procedures, but with care to not spread the radioactive material around (**Fig. 18**). The skin around the laceration may be wiped off to ensure contamination is not washed into the wound. Often the normal procedure for flushing a laceration is to drape with surgical towels to catch runoff. In this case, we will limit the runoff of contaminated water by using disposable absorbant underpads underneath the normal draping. The edges of the drapes are taped down to try to keep runoff from getting under the drapes. It is often difficult to make an absolute watertight seal at the edge of the drapes. In **Fig. 19** we use absorbent pads to catch the runoff as soon as it leaves the laceration. As soon as a pad becomes saturated, the flushing should be paused while new dry pads are put in place. If time permits, the draping, taping, and collection of runoff in a garbage can will help control

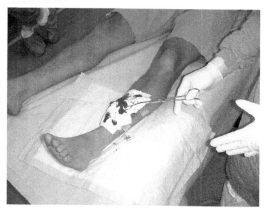

Fig. 16. Dressing removal.

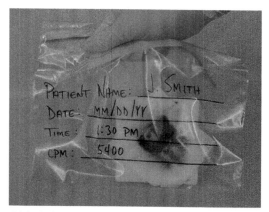

Fig. 17. Bagged and labeled wound dressing.

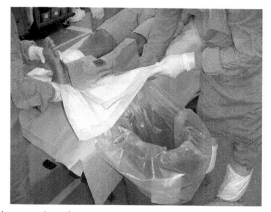

Fig. 18. Wound drape and catch can.

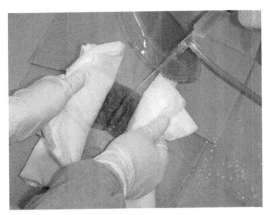

Fig. 19. Catch wound flush with ABD pads.

contamination. However, the primary method for containing the flush water is the use of an assistant to catch the runoff in absorbent abdominal (ABD) pads. The chances of removing contamination are greatest on the first washings so flush easily. Avoiding aggressive flushing may limit the spread of contamination. Remember that flushing and manipulation of wounds can be painful, so medicine always comes first. Administration of pain medication as ordered, and injectable lidocaine may be used.

After flushing, blot with a 4 × 4 gauze (**Fig. 20**). Blot once and throw away and then get a new pad to blot once again. Repeated dabbing with the same 4 × 4 may spread contamination around. Then cover the open wound as you remove and discard the drapes into contaminated trash. Clean pads are placed under the limb and a second survey or wound count is done to document the progress made with the decontamination efforts (**Fig. 21**).

The reduction in count rate is documented in the nursing note and the decontamination procedure is repeated. A decrease in counts indicates contamination is being removed. Our goal is to flush until clean or as clean as we can get it. Is remaining activity dangerous? To determine this, medicine needs to integrate with health physics. If

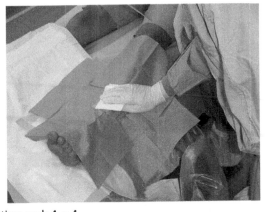

Fig. 20. Blot one time each 4 × 4.

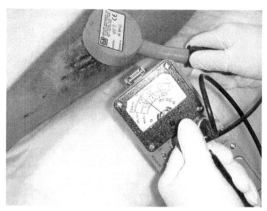

Fig. 21. Second wound count.

the material is a gamma emitter, the situation may be different than if an alpha emitter is detected. Health Physics support can advise if further efforts, including surgical debridement, are necessary. Otherwise, the decision to suture is based on wound healing and infection control. These considerations highlight the need to identify the material and whether it is an alpha, beta, or gamma emitter. Absent your own resource person, REAC/TS is on call 24/7.

During the survey, an area of contamination was found on the patient's chest (**Fig. 22**). The person with the meter can show the patient care team where the contamination is located or mark the area with a surgical marking pen. This is a handy technique for remembering where multiple areas of contamination were found or if there are multiple patients being surveyed. There is no rush about decontaminating intact skin. The skin is an effective barrier against most radioactive contaminants.[26] If the patient complains of burning or irritation, it indicates chemical or thermal processes, not radiation. If that is the case, then the ED team needs to flush immediately following normal chemical decontamination protocols. Remember, chemical contamination may represent an immediate threat to the patient and the ED caregivers. Straightforward contamination with radioactive material does not.

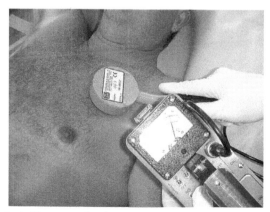

Fig. 22. Finding intact skin contamination.

One of the best and most-simple methods for cleaning skin is a simple premoistened wipe (**Fig. 23**). The area is cleaned in an outside to inside manner. Think of cleaning up a paint spill. A useful trick for more stubborn skin contamination is seen in **Fig. 24**. Place an absorbent material over the contamination and then cover and seal with a plastic material. A large IV Op Site or plastic wrap works to seal the area. After 3 or 4 hours, the skin will sweat the material into the absorbent pad. Be sure to use the absorbent pad underneath the plastic to prevent forming a pool of contaminated sweat. If necessary, the area can be draped in the manner shown earlier for a wound cleanse. A soapy 4 × 4 or soft scrubbing pad could be used to clean a little harder. Hopefully, the area will become clean, but be careful not to irritate the skin, as this could increase the intake of radioactive material.

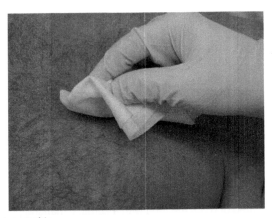

Fig. 23. Cleaning intact skin.

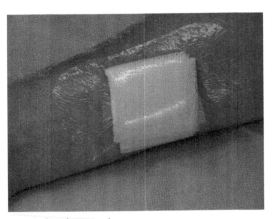

Fig. 24. Plastic wrap and absorbent pad.

Before the patient leaves the ED to be admitted or discharged, a final survey is performed. Any wounds with persistent contamination may be wrapped to contain that contamination. If the patient is not ambulatory, we log roll the patient again and be sure the patient is lying on a clean sheet. Then a complete radiological survey, head to toe, front and back, slowly and carefully should be completed (**Fig. 25**). The patient can go to the floor by stretcher or wheel chair, whichever is appropriate (**Fig. 26**). If ambulatory, the patient could stand for the final survey like anyone else leaving the area.

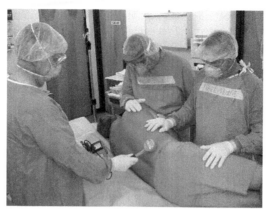

Fig. 25. Final survey.

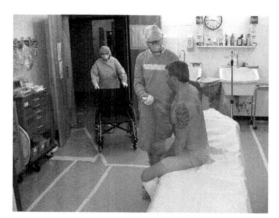

Fig. 26. Discharge.

Patients should be admitted to the hospital based on their medical needs. It is certainly possible that a patient could be admitted to the appropriate medical department with some remaining contamination present. Patients should not be held in the ED when they need to be transferred to appropriate continuing care. All departments and staff need to understand the basics of radiation exposure and radioactive contamination so they too realize that these situations are not difficult to handle. If the patient's medical condition does not require admission, remaining areas of contamination may be covered and the patient referred to appropriate follow-up for decontamination issues. The purpose of the ED is to take care of hurt people. Being contaminated is not a reason to keep someone out who needs treatment. Likewise, uninjured patients who are only contaminated have no reason to be seen in the ED.

When the patient has left the area, it is time for the caregivers to remove their protective clothing and leave. This clothing is usually removed in a head-to-toe sequence, leaving the face mask on until the last step before removing inner gloves and shoe covers and stepping across the control line. All employees are surveyed head to toe before going to other areas unless medical emergencies require their presence immediately. Likewise, the treatment area should be surveyed clean before other use, unless an emergency exists. Remember, lifesaving always comes before concerns over simple radioactive contamination.

The information presented is based on sound principles, but is not to be taken as an absolute standard for decontamination. For instance, in a multipatient scenario, someone with a simple laceration on the forearm might have the area flushed and covered and then be kept in a holding area while more serious patients are seen.

Remember the basic points.

- Medical priorities always come first.
- Radioactive contamination can be dealt with using little more than normal trauma or biological precautions. Consider airway precautions.
- The objective is to deliver proper patient care while trying to contain the contamination.
- Ensure there is no chemical threat. Often the chemical nature of the material is more dangerous than the fact that it is radioactive. Chemical threats require chemical precautions.
- A survey meter should be available and staff trained to use it.
- Time: Reducing time exposed reduces dose.
- Distance: If not involved in immediate patient care, take a step back.
- Reduce quantity: As soon as possible, remove the patient's contaminated clothing carefully and double bag out of the area.
- Identify the specific radioactive nuclide as soon as possible.
- The patient contaminated only with radioactive material only does not represent a serious threat to caregivers if properly handled with basic alterations in nursing care.
- More detailed education on radiation emergencies is available at the REAC/TS Web site. Classes are available from REAC/TS by calling 865-576-3131 or at https://orise.orau.gov/reacts/

REFERENCES

1. Mihai L, Milu C, Voicu B, et al. Ionizing radiation, understanding and acceptance. Health Phys 2005;89(4):375–82.
2. Ashley Fantz C. For Ebola caregivers, enormous fear, risk and bravery - CNN.com. Atlanta (GA): CNN; 2016. Available at: http://www.cnn.com/2014/10/12/health/ebola-health-care-workers/. Accessed February 29, 2016.
3. Smithson A. History of sarin attack and analysis of lessons learned. Washington, DC: Stimson Think Tank; 2016. p. 71–2. Available at: http://www.stimson.org/images/uploads/research-pdfs/atxchapter3.pdf. Accessed March 7, 2016.
4. REAC/TS Registry of Radiation Incidents. REAC/TS registry. Oak Ridge (TN): Radiation Emergency Assistance Center/Training Site; 2016.
5. Delves D, Fllitton S, editors. The radiological accident in Goiana. Vienna (Australia): IAEA; 1988. p. 23–7.
6. Bandeira De, Carvalho A. The psychological impact of the radiological accident in goiania. In: International seminar recovery operations in the event of a nuclear accident or radiological emergency, 21. Rio de Janeiro (Brazil): National Nuclear Energy Commission; 1989. p. 19. Available at: http://www.iaea.org/inis/collection/NCLCollectionStore/_Public/20/008/20008221.pdf. Accessed February 29, 2016.
7. Carvalho A. The psychological impact of the radiological accident in Goiana. Vienna (Australia): IAEA; 1989. p. 468.
8. Mettler F, Upton A. Medical effects of ionizing radiation. Philadelphia: Saunders/Elsevier; 2008. p. 8.

9. NCRP, Staff, M, National Council on Radiation Protection. Ionizing radiation exposure of the population of the United States: recommendations of the National Council on Radiation Protection and Measurements. 160th edition. 2009.

10. NCRP. Management of persons accidentally contaminated with radionuclides. Bethesda (MD): National Council On Radiation Protection and Measurements; 1980. p. 44.

11. Baes F. hps.org. Health Physics Society. 2016. Available at: http://hps.org/publicinformation/ate/faqs/radiationtypes.html. Accessed May 5, 2016.

12. Ansari A. Radiation threats and your safety: a guide to preparation and response for professionals and community. Boca Raton (FL): Chapman & Hall/CRC; 2009. p. 30.

13. Gollnick D. Basic radiation protection technology. Altadena (CA): Pacific Radiation Corp; 2011.

14. Sugarman S, Goans R, Garrett S, et al. The medical aspects of radiation incidents. Radiation Emergency Assistance Center/Training Site. 2016. p. 8. Available at: https://orise.orau.gov/files/reacts/medical-aspects-of-radiation-incidents.pdf. Accessed May 5, 2016.

15. Department of Homeland Security Medical Preparedness and Response Subgroup. Department of Homeland Security Working Group on Radiological Dispersal Device (RDD) preparedness. Washington, DC: Department of Homeland Security; 2003. p. 29.

16. NRC. Information for radiation workers. Rockville (MD): Nuclear Regulatory Commission; 2016. Available at: http://www.nrc.gov/about-nrc/radiation/health-effects/info.html. Accessed February 29, 2016.

17. Industrial Radiography | Radiation Protection | US EPA. Environmental Protection Agency. 2016. Available at: http://www.epa.gov/rpdweb01/industrial-radiography.html. Accessed February 29, 2016.

18. Radiation Protection | US EPA. Environmental Protection Agency. 2016. Available at: http://www.epa.gov/radiation/sources/food_irrad.html. Accessed February 29, 2016.

19. Irradiation facility Oin Nesvizh. Vienna (Austria): IAEA; 1996.

20. About Lymphocyte Depletion Kinetics - Radiation Emergency Medical Management. Remmnlmgov. 2016. Available at: http://www.remm.nlm.gov/aboutlymphocytedepletion.htm. Accessed February 29, 2016.

21. Ricks R, Berger M, O'Hara F. The medical basis for radiation-accident preparedness. Boca Raton (FL): Parthenon Pub. Group; 2002. p. 11–22.

22. Generic procedures for medical response during a nuclear or radiological emergency. Vienna (Austria): IAEA; 2005. p. 17.

23. Paull J, Rosenthal F. Heat strain and heat stress for workers wearing protective suits at a hazardous waste site. Am Ind Hyg Assoc J 1987;48(5):458–63. Available at: http://www.ncbi.nlm.nih.gov/pubmed/3591668. Accessed February 29, 2016.

24. Respiratory Protection. – CFR 1910.134. Occupational Safety and Health Administration. 2016. Available at: https://www.osha.gov/pls/oshaweb/owadisp.show_document?p_table=standards&p_id=12716. Accessed February 29, 2016.

25. ATLS Advanced Trauma Life Support for Doctors - student course manual. 9th edition. Chicago: American College of Surgeons Committee on Trauma; 2012. p. 6–7.

26. Borron S, Kazzi Z. Management of hazardous material emergencies. Emerg Med Clin North Am 2015;33(1):xvii.

Vehicle of Hope

Faith-based Disaster Response

Deborah J. Persell, PhD, RN, APN

KEYWORDS

- Hurricane Katrina • Faith-based disaster response • Hope • Herth Hope Index
- Phenomenology • Mixed methods

KEY POINTS

- Faith-based disaster response engages in the work of hope.
- The Herth Hope Index is a valid and reliable measure of hope for those doing the work of or receiving benefit of the work of faith-based disaster response.
- The work of faith-based disaster response can be a vehicle of hope.

In August 2005, the United States experienced one of the most catastrophic and costly disasters in its history: Hurricane Katrina. Few were affected more than those living in New Orleans. In the 10 plus years since, much has been written regarding the whole of the response. Most agree Faith-based Organizations (FBOs) made a major contribution to the response and recovery efforts.[1,2] Faith-based disaster response includes nurses as staff, volunteers, and recipients of services. Whereas activities and skill sets of FBOs vary, similar core missions exist: to provide hope. Many of the FBOs were registered with the National Volunteer Organizations Active in Disaster (NVOAD), the official organization designated by the National Response Plan to represent non-government organizations. The FBO-registered names with NVOAD reflect their mission of hope: Convoy of Hope, Restoring or Restores Hope (multiple agencies), Hope Animal Assistance Crisis Response, Hope Coalition of America, Hope Worldwide, Sharing Hope in Crisis, and HopeForce International.[3] The purpose of this article is to expand understanding of "hope" in the context of disaster response.

Conflict of Interest: The author has no commercial or financial conflicts of interest to disclose. There is no funding source for this research.

Regional Center for Disaster Preparedness Education, College of Nursing and Health Professions, Arkansas State University, 105 North Caraway, PO Box 910, State University (Jonesboro), AR 72467, USA

E-mail address: dpersell@astate.edu

CONCEPT OF HOPE

As a concept, hope has been purported to be essential for health and well-being.[4] It is viewed as multidimensional,[5] a life force,[6] and highly individualized.[7] Antecedents of hope include stress, loss, despair, and threats to life. Outcomes associated with hope include coping, peace, and an elevated quality of life.[4] Hope has been studied as an intervention.[8] Others find hope as a result of interventions[6,9] that assist individuals in developing a plan for the future and developing goals.[10] The long-term impact of hope has been studied.[9]

Valid and reliable tools exist to measure hope, as shown in **Table 1**. The theoretic framework is similar among them and found in related bodies of literature.[6,11] The brief 12-item Herth Hope Index (HHI) was chosen for this study because its spiritual component is complementary to the study's context.

METHODOLOGY

This mixed methods study used phenomenology-based interviews and the HHI. The Institutional Review Board approved the research. Informed consent was obtained from each participant. Data collection occurred 2 years after Hurricane Katrina. Forty-two participants in 26 interviews, connected to the faith-based response in New Orleans, responded to the following question: "What stands out to you about your experience receiving assistance from, being staff with, or volunteering with faith-based disaster response?" All interviews were recorded and transcribed by the researcher. For this article, a secondary analysis related to hope has been performed using 22 of the transcribed interviews. This study also includes 4 group volunteer interviews analyzed for the first time. Themes for the analysis are the HHI items. The qualitative software package nVivo was used to assist with data analysis. Results of the HHI were scored and entered into SPSS for analysis. Triangulated findings yielded a comprehensive analysis of hope in faith-based disaster response.

SAMPLE

A convenience sample was recruited from one FBO active in New Orleans for 2 years after Katrina: 28 volunteers, 9 staff, and 5 residents. A preponderance of the volunteers and staff were men with most of the residents being women. All of the volunteers and staff, except 1, were Caucasian (1 was a Pacific Islander). All residents were African American. Volunteers and staff represented a range of ages (22–73 years of age); residents were 40 to 59 years of age, as shown in **Table 2**. Volunteers and staff came from 11 states. New Orleans was home to all residents. Most participants were married. More than half of the volunteers had annual incomes greater than $50,000. Two-thirds of the staff had annual incomes of $25,001 to $50,000. All residents had annual incomes less than $50,000. All of the volunteers and staff had completed high school with the vast majority having a college education. Only one resident had completed high school; the others did not.

QUANTITATIVE FINDINGS

Results of the HHI are the quantitative data. Descriptive statistics, analysis of variance, and correlation tests were performed. Individual responses were scored per the index instructions; items 3 and 6 were reverse scored. The maximum possible score is 48. Group total scores are reported in **Fig. 1**.

With P at .05, item analysis of the HHI items reveals no statistical difference between groups for 10 of 12 items. When the post-hoc Levine Statistic is used, statistical

Table 1
Comparison of Literatures on Measurements of Hope

Hope Scale	Theoretical Underpinning	Sample	Number of Items	Cronbach's Alpha for Total Scale	Cronbach's Alpha for Subscales	Test-Retest	Content Validity	Construct Validity
Miller Hope Scale,[33] 1988	Dufault, Korner, Lynch and Marcel	75 university students	40	Pre-test = .95		2-week .87	4 judges with expertise in area of hope	6 experts in measurement
		522 university students	40	.93				Correlations with Psychological Well-being scale r = .71 Existential Well-being Scale r = .82 Hopelessness Scale r = -.54
Nowotny Hope Scale,[34] 1989	Frankl, Dufault, Hinds, Miller and Powers, Lazarus and others	306 adults with cancer or experienced stressful event	47	.90	Six subscales with range of .60 to .90	Not Reported	Panel of six experts	Correlation with Beck's Hopelessness Scale r = -.47
Herth Hope Scale,[35] 1991	Dufault & Martocchio	20 Cancer support group	32	Pre-test = .84	Factor I = .89 Factor II = .85 Factor III = .84	3-week .89 to .91	4 judges with expertise in hope	Factor analysis with varimax rotation explained 52% of the variance
		40 Oncology sample	32	Pilot test = .75				Correlation with Beck's Hopelessness Scale r = -.69
		120 Cancer patients	32	.89				
		185 well adults	30	.92	Factor I = .91			
		40 elderly	30	.94	Factor II = .90			
		75 Bereaved elderly	30	.95	Factor III = .87			

(continued on next page)

Table 1
(continued)

Hope Scale	Theoretical Underpinning	Sample	Number of Items	Cronbach's Alpha for Total Scale	Cronbach's Alpha for Subscales	Test-Retest	Content Validity	Construct Validity
Herth Hope Index,[36] 1992		20 physically ill adults 172 adults: 70 acute 71 chronic 31 terminal	12 12	Pilot test = .94 .97 .98 .96 .94	Range of .78 to .86	3-week .89 to .91	Two judges for construct validity and 12 for face validity	*Factor analysis with varimax rotation explained 52% of the variance* Correlations with Existential Well-Being Scale r = .78 Nowotny Hope Scale r = .89 Hopelessness Scale r = −.47
Multi-dimensional Hope Scale,[37] 1994	Dufault, Engel, Farber, French, Herth, Korner, Lewin, Lynch, McGee, Menninger, and Stotland	56 adults with chronic illness 450 adults with chronic illness	Modified Stoner Hope Scale 49	Pilot test not reported 95	Factor I = .85 Factor II = .85 Factor III = .92 Factor IV = .85 Factor V = .77 Factor VI = .88	Not Reported	Two hope content specialists Inter-rater reliability of 0.85	Inter-item correlations ranged from r = .03 to r = .84 Correlated with Beck's Hopelessness Scale r = −.40
Snyder Hope Scale,[38] 1995	Stotland, Averill, First, Seligman, and Bandura	Reported as 1000+, but did not cite specific study 1,025 individuals between 16-70 who had been admitted to the hospital for trauma care 27 individuals 60 tumor free oral cancer patients	12 8 (four distractor items are omitted) 8 (four distractor items are omitted) 12	Range of .74 to .84 .84 .76 .81	.74 to .84 .81 for agency items .80 for pathways items Not reported .76 for pathways items .70 for agency items	3-10 weeks >.80 Not reported Not reported	Not explicitly identified	Not explicitly identified

Scale	Theorists	Sample	No. of items	Internal consistency	Reliability	Test-retest	Factor structure	Validity
(Snyder's) State Hope Scale,[39] 1996	Schachtel, Stotland, Menninger, Frankl, Beck, Weissman, Lester, Lee, Locke, Latham, and Pervin, among others	Pilot study = 444 adults 27 individuals	8 6	.82 to .95 median .93 (data collected daily over 30 days) .92 (median overall value)	Range of .83 to .95 with median .91 for agency items and .74 to .93 with median .91 for pathways items Not reported	Not reported	Not explicitly identified	(rs for days 1 and 29 respectively) Correlations with Dispositional Hope Scale rs =.79 and .78 State Self-Esteem Scale rs =.68 and .75 State Positive Affect Schedule rs=.65 and .55 State Negative Affect Schedule rs = –.47 and –.50
(Snyder's) Children's Hope Scale,[40] 1997	Dweck, Barker, Dembo, Lewin, Kliewer, Lewis, Rutter, Werner, & Smith	Pilot study = 372 42 adolescents with Type 1 Diabetes 313 students from public high schools 356 students from public middle schools	12 6 6 6 6	.74 .77 .88 .84 .83	.72 to .86 Not reported Not reported	One month .81 One month .71 to .73 Not reported	Not explicitly identified	Confirmatory factor analysis yielded GFI = .96 and CFI = .95, supported two-factor model Correlations with Child Depression Inventory r = –.48 Global self-worth index of the Self-Perception Profile for Children r = .52 Student's Life Satisfaction Scale r = .55 Child and Adolescent Social Support Scale r = .53

(continued on next page)

Table 1 (continued)

Hope Scale	Theoretical Underpinning	Sample	Number of Items	Cronbach's Alpha for Total Scale	Cronbach's Alpha for Subscales	Test-Retest	Content Validity	Construct Validity
Snyder Hope Scale (Hebrew),[41] 2002	See original SHS	60 adults: 53 with schizophrenia 7 with schizoaffective disorder	12	.80		Not reported	Not explicitly identified	Not explicitly identified
		179 adults with diagnosis of a severe mental illness	12	.80	.71 for pathways items .76 for agency items			
Miller Hope Scale,[42] 2005	Concept development, multiple theoretical stances	1036 7th & 8th graders	40	.92	Satisfaction with life = .91 Avoidance of Hope Threats = .83 Anticipation of a Future = .76	Not Reported	Inter-rater reliability of .88	Confirmatory factor analysis yielding a Cronbach's alpha of .93 and a subscale alpha range of .75 to .82 Subsequent recommendation to reduce scale: 13 item hope scale and 9 item hopelessness scale
Children's Hope Scale (Portuguese),[43] 2009	See original CHS	Pilot study = 42 students	6	.74			Not explicitly identified	Not explicitly identified
		367 6th–8th grade students		.81	.55 to .64	One year .51		
Herth Hope Scale (Spanish),[44] 2010		315 college students	29 (item 29 removed)	.89	Optimism/social support = .81 Hopelessness = .78 Agency = .77 Social-Support/ Belonging = .73	Not reported	Authors performed content validity post-translation Backward-forward translation procedure	Factor analysis with promax rotation explained 38.6% of total variance

Scale	Authors	Sample		Reliability	Subscale reliability	Test-retest	Translation	Validity
Locus-of-Hope Scale (extension of SHS),[45] 2010	Snyder, Bandura, Briones, Tolentino, Markus and Kitayama, Miller	Pilot study 1 = 210 college students ages 16-23	40	Not reported	Internal = .80 External-family = .91 External-peers = .87 External-spiritual = .95	Not reported	Not explicitly identified	Confirmatory factor analysis yielding Cronbach's alpha range of .80 to .95 for subscales
		Pilot study 2 = 268 college students ages 16-21	40	Not reported	Subscales range from .69-.91			Confirmatory factory analysis yielding RMSEA = .049, CFI = .91, TLI = .91
		1,008 college students	40	Not reported	Subscales range from .80-.96			
Herth Hope Index (Dutch),[46] 2010	Dufault & Martocchio	Pilot study = 25	12	Not reported	Not reported	One-week .79	Backward-forward translation procedure	Principal Component Analysis with varimax rotation explained 47% of the variance. Correlates with Manchester Short Assessment of Quality of Life $r = .56$ Loneliness Scale $r = -.47$
		341	12	.84				
Integrative Hope Scale,[47] 2011	Snyder, Miller, Herth	Pilot study = 489 individuals aged ≥ 16	23	.92	Trust and confidence = .85 Lack of perspective = .85 Positive future orientation = .80 Social relations and personal value = .85	Not reported	Backward-forward translation procedure	Correlations with Miller Hope scale $r = .73$ to .92 Herth Hope Index $r = .64$ to .81 Allgemeine Depressionsskala = −.58 Dimensions intercorrelate between $r = .52$ and .63
		200 adults with schizophrenia or schizoaffective disorder	22	.92	.78 to .86	2-week overall .84; subscales .71 to .83		

Herth Hope Index (Chinese),[48] 2012	Dufault & Martocchio	120 patients with heart failure	12	.89	Range of .76 to .88	Two-week .86 Subscales range from .72 to .81	Backward-forward translation procedure	Correlations with Rosenberg Self-Esteem Scale $r = .4$ Hamilton Depression Rating Scale $r = -.4$
Herth Hope Index (Italian),[49] 2012		266 cancer patients	12	.84	Not reported	Two-week .64	Backward-forward translation procedure	Confirmatory factor analysis yielded CFI of .91, TLI of .91 and RMSEA of .06 Correlates with FACIT spiritual well-being scale $r = .68$ Hospital Anxiety and Depression Scale $r = -.51$
Children's Hope Scale-Peabody Treatment Progress Battery (PTPB),[50] 2012	See original CHS	Pilot study = 213 youth receiving mental health treatment	4	.87	.72 to .82	Not reported	Not explicitly identified	Correlates with original Children's Hope Scale with $r = .97$

Abbreviations: CFI, comparative fit index; CHS, children's hope scale; FACIT, functional assessment of chronic illness therapy [scale]; GFI, goodness of fit index; RMSEA, root mean square error of approximation; SHS, snyder hope scale; TLI, tucker lewis index.

Table 2
Sample demographics

Demographic	Volunteers	Residents	Staff
Gender			
Male	19	1	6
Female	9	4	3
Age			
22–29	6	0	1
30–39	1	0	2
40–49	6	2	1
50–59	6	3	1
60–69	7	0	4
70–73	2	0	0
Marital status			
Single	3	1	0
Married	24	3	9
Divorced	1	1	0
Ethnicity			
White	27	0	0
African American	0	5	9
Pacific Islander	1	0	0
Education			
Did not graduate high school	0	4	0
GED or diploma	6	1	2
College	22	0	7
Annual income			
Under $10,000	1	0	0
$10,001–$25,000	1	2	0
$25,001–$50,000	10	3	6
$50,001–$75,000	7	0	0
Over $75,000	9	0	3
State of residence			
Missouri	5	0	0
Kansas	2	0	0
Oklahoma	8	0	0
Ohio	6	0	3
Michigan	2	0	1
Massachusetts	3	0	0
North Carolina	1	0	1
New Hampshire	1	0	0
Louisiana	0	5	2
Idaho	0	0	1
Oregon	0	0	1

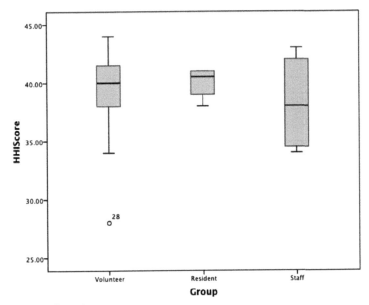

Fig. 1. HHI scores box plot.

significance is found (0.014) between the volunteers and staff on the item "I feel my life has value and worth." Statistical significance is also found (0.046) between volunteers and residents for the item "I can see possibilities in the midst of difficulties." The Cronbach α for this study, based on standardized items, is 0.705. Complete results for item responses can be found in **Table 3**.

Interitem correlation is demonstrated. The only strong correlation (0.762) was between "I believe that each day has potential" and "I feel my life has value and worth." Moderate correlations are evident as follows:

I have a positive outlook toward life
I have short- and/or long-range goals: 0.642
I have a faith that gives me comfort: 0.405
I believe that each day has potential: 0.450
I can see possibilities in the midst of difficulties
I have a faith that gives me comfort: 0.522
I have deep inner strength: 0.484
I have a faith that gives me comfort
I have deep inner strength: 0.562
I can recall happy/joyful times
I am able to give and receive caring/love: 0.417
I have a sense of direction: 0.431
I believe each day has potential: 0.499
I feel my life has value and worth: 0.429
I have a sense of direction
I am able to give and receive caring/love: 0.528
I believe each day has potential: 0.646
I feel my life has value and worth: 0.578
I believe that each day has potential

Table 3
Herth Hope Index item results

Item	Group Volunteer	Resident	Staff	Total
I have a positive outlook toward life.				
Strongly disagree	1	0	0	1
Disagree	1	0	0	1
Agree	10	1	3	14
Strongly agree	16	4	5	25
I feel all alone.				
Strongly disagree	17	4	5	26
Disagree	11	1	3	15
Agree	0	0	0	0
Strongly agree	0	0	0	0
I can see possibilities in the midst of difficulties.				
Strongly disagree	0	1	0	1
Disagree	0	0	0	0
Agree	17	3	5	25
Strongly agree	11	1	3	15
I have a faith that gives me comfort.				
Strongly disagree	1	1	0	2
Disagree	0	0	0	0
Agree	1	0	1	2
Strongly agree	25	4	6	35
I feel scared about my future.				
Strongly disagree	14	4	3	21
Disagree	10	1	3	14
Agree	2	0	2	4
Strongly agree	1	0	0	1
I have short- and/or long-range goals.				
Strongly disagree	1	0	0	1
Disagree	0	0	0	0
Agree	13	1	2	16
Strongly agree	14	4	6	24
I can recall happy/joyful times.				
Strongly disagree	0	0	0	0
Disagree	0	0	0	0
Agree	7	1	3	11
Strongly agree	21	4	5	30
I have deep inner strength.				
Strongly disagree	0	1	0	1
Disagree	0	0	0	0
Agree	13	0	3	16
Strongly agree	15	4	5	24

(continued on next page)

Table 3
(continued)

Item	Volunteer	Resident	Staff	Total
		Group		
I am able to give and receive caring/love.				
Strongly disagree	0	0	0	0
Disagree	0	0	0	0
Agree	10	0	4	14
Strongly agree	18	5	4	27
I have a sense of direction.				
Strongly disagree	0	0	0	0
Disagree	0	0	0	0
Agree	10	2	5	17
Strongly agree	18	3	3	24
I believe that each day has potential.				
Strongly disagree	0	0	0	0
Disagree	0	0	0	0
Agree	3	1	4	8
Strongly agree	25	4	4	33
I feel my life has value and worth.				
Strongly disagree	0	0	0	0
Disagree	0	0	0	0
Agree	3	1	4	8
Strongly agree	25	4	4	33

I feel my life has value and worth: 0.762
I feel my life has value and worth
I am able to give and receive caring/love: 0.414

Multiple weak correlations are demonstrated but not reported here.
As items 3 and 6 were reverse scored, the negative correlations were expected:
Item no. 3, Feeling all alone, had the most frequent negative correlations:

I have a positive outlook toward life: -0.404
I have short- and/or long-range goals: -0.343
I can see possibilities in the midst of difficulties: -0.090
I have a faith that gives me comfort: -0.106
I can recall happy/joyful times: -0.332
I have deep inner strength: -0.201
I have a sense of direction: -0.256
I believe that each day has potential: -0.353
I feel my life has value and worth: -0.180

Item no. 6, I feel scared about my future, had fewer and weaker negative correlations and are as follows:

I have a positive outlook toward life: -0.262
I can recall happy/joyful times: -0.036
I am able to give and receive caring/love: -0.235

I have a sense of direction: −0.230
I believe that each day has potential: −0.340
I feel my life has value and worth: −0.106

QUALITATIVE FINDINGS

Participant interviews are the qualitative data. To reduce bias, the researcher submitted to a bracketing interview. Member checking was performed for the original study but not the secondary analysis.

The word hope is referenced in every interview and occurs 229 times, representing 0.27% of the interview content, as shown in **Figs. 2–5**. Hope is 44th in the most frequent 100 words of all interviews. The word is always spoken as a reference implying that researcher knows what hope means. A frequent phrase in the interviews is "they [it] gave me hope." One staff participant offered a definition of hope in a very spiritual context:

It's the absolute confidence that everything's going to be just fine. Even though at times it might be hard, that confidence is still there, it's still that halo hanging there, that reassurance that everything is going to be fine.

My only idea of hope is that hope is walking with the Lord. Probably the most quoted scripture of all time is Jeremiah 20:11; not exactly New Orleans, but of truly battered people being told that the Lord has all of the plans for the future laid out for you, plans to give you hope. If the Lord has everything laid out for your future that means hope is the Lord, hope is in the Lord.

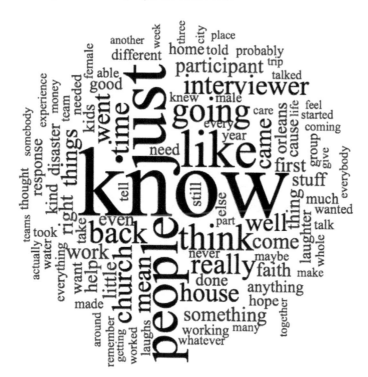

Fig. 2. Most frequent 100 words.

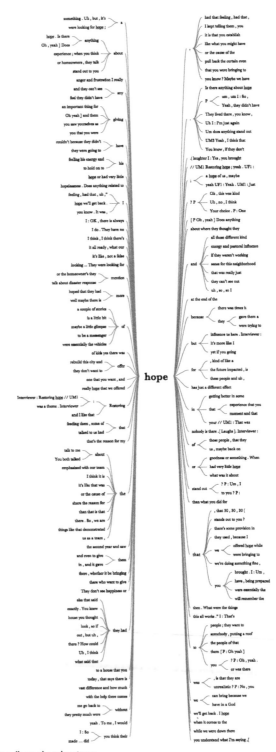

Fig. 3. Word Tree (hope) volunteer.

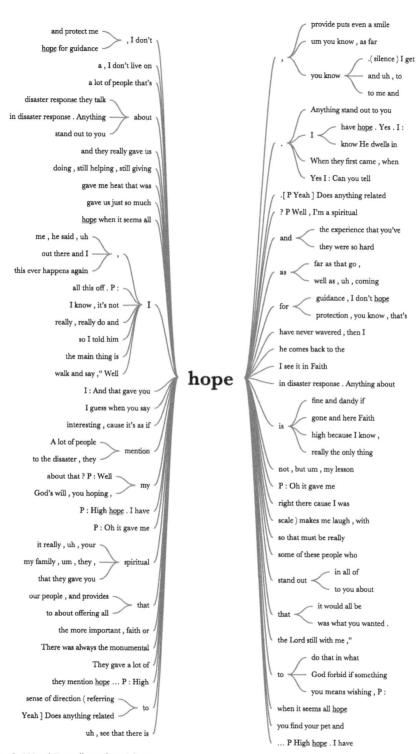

Fig. 4. Word Tree (hope) residents.

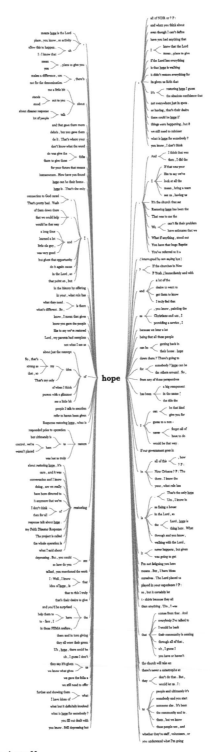

Fig. 5. Word Tree (hope) staff.

There are limited references (18 in 5 interviews) to having no hope or feeling hopeless. Not one reference to hopelessness is found in the resident's interviews. Hopelessness is always in the context of staff or volunteers projecting it on the situation in New Orleans with the caveat that, although the situation seemed hopeless, the people did not

Volunteer A: Utter hopelessness for the people down there. Just, I just couldn't believe all the devastation and how it must have upset their lives, probably forever, and I just felt what little bit I was going to do wasn't going to help the whole area. I just felt utter hopelessness.

Volunteer B: We both have been in situations before that we think should be hopeless but the people aren't...

Staff: They're sitting there hopeless. Does God really care? And then, all these people show up.

Data to support items on the HHI are presented in **Table 4**.

The first HHI item is "I have a positive outlook toward life." A total of 125 references to this statement are found in 22 interviews, including all residents and staff and 11 of 12 volunteer interviews. The most references are from the residents of New Orleans. Data or reference samples supporting this item include the following:

Volunteer: We can see that things are still good; maybe not for them, life is really bad, but there is something better going on...

Resident: Think about what you can do to uplift someone, encourage someone else, and He [the Lord] is going to provide for me. So, I'm going to be blessed regardless... Because I know this, I'm going to do what I can to get in that house as I go along, and I get a lot of enjoyment from that.

Staff: They just roofed the wrong house... no excuse for it. No excuse. But, the homeowner pulled into the driveway and saw that the house was roofed. They were just so discouraged that they were coming home to commit suicide and when they saw the new roof on their house that changed their outlook on life completely.

The second HHI item is "I have short- and/or long-range goals." Of 12 volunteer interviews, 9 contain references, as did 3 of 5 resident interviews and 5 of 9 staff interviews. A total of 17 interviews, containing 33 references, support this item. Examples of data for this item are as follows:

Volunteer: We told them [staff] when we got down there, "You're down here serving the people of New Orleans; we're down here to serve you."

Resident: I just wanted to show them some southern hospitality. I had baked beans made and was serving them red beans for lunch. Some of the groups hadn't had crayfish and I introduced them to crayfish; I wanted to show my gratitude like that.

Staff: They have started bringing back community members to roles filled by volunteers. So, it was a healthy transition because outsiders shouldn't have to fill those roles. It was a nice passage, changing of the guard.

The third HHI item is "I feel all alone" with 19 interviews and 62 references. Eight of interviews and 23 references are from volunteers, 4 interviews with 17 references from residents, and 7 interviews with 22 references from the staff. Data samples include the following:

Volunteer: It just felt so lost down there and people were like, everyone's forgotten about us, the whole country has forgotten.

Table 4
References coded to Herth Hope Index items

Item	Interviews 12 Volunteer with 29 Participants	5 Resident	9 Staff	Total 26
I have a positive outlook toward life.				
No. of interviews	11	5	9	25
No. of references	43	43	35	125
I have short- and/or long-range goals.				
No. of interviews	9	3	5	17
No. of references	17	4	12	33
I feel all alone.				
No. of interviews	8	4	7	19
No. of references	23	17	22	62
I can see possibilities in the midst of difficulties.				
No. of interviews	7	5	2	14
No. of references	11	8	2	21
I have a faith that gives me comfort.				
No. of interviews	9	4	9	22
No. of references	34	48	63	145
I feel scared about my future.				
No. of interviews	8	4	7	19
No. of references	34	16	25	75
I can recall happy/joyful times.				
No. of interviews	10	5	7	22
No. of references	23	16	18	57
I have deep inner strength.				
No. of interviews	7	5	5	17
No. of references	15	11	14	40
I am able to give and receive caring/love.				
No. of interviews	9	5	9	23
No. of references	19	56	70	145
I have a sense of direction.				
No. of interviews	11	5	9	25
No. of references	56	26	64	146
I believe that each day has potential.				
No. of interviews	6	4	4	14
No. of references	7	6	8	21
I feel my life has value and worth.				
No. of interviews	11	4	8	23
No. of references	52	40	62	154

Resident: My sister said Mama was on the coast, just crying, saying, "My whole family is gone" because her three sisters were in there (in the house with the 22 people). Mama said, "I'm all alone, I'm all alone, all my whole family is gone."

Staff: And then there's this little, this little ghost town. And over here, there's probably a couple but you see that little ghost town and that little ghost town and there's nothing there. This is a place where people live and there's not a person in sight. It's sunk! Drive on down the road and nobody, there's a church over here and nobody there, no people. And I am depressed.

The fourth HHI item "I can see possibilities in the midst of difficulties" is supported in 14 interviews with 21 references. This item includes 7 volunteer interviews with 11 references, 5 resident interviews with 8 references, and 2 staff interviews with 2 references. Data include the following:

Volunteer: …gave them a place to start rather than coming back and saying I don't know where to start. Now, it's all cleaned out so I can start by putting it back together again now.

Resident: I'm just so anxious to get in. I'm excited, I'm excited about being able to get in the kitchen and be able to cook again, not having to go to the Laundromat and being able to just spread out a little bit so I won't be so cramped. I'm just really excited about all of that.

Staff: …he was too choked up and took this paper and he had one of the boys read it. It was the notice to FEMA to take that house off the destruction list; he and his wife had prayed it through the night before, after having dinner with them [the boys], and they were going to rebuild the house.

The fifth HHI item is "I have a faith that gives me comfort." Twenty-two interviews contain 145 references: 9 volunteer interviews with 34 references, 4 resident interviews with 48 references, and 9 staff interviews with 63 references. Samples of those data follow:

Volunteer: To experience firsthand being a servant, how rewarding that can be to other people and even to you. It was a great blessing to us; we tried to make it about other people but I couldn't help myself sensing God's presence there, going out to these people in need and it's almost like I got to go do this; I got to go be with Him; I've got to go join Him in what He's doing.

Resident: I'm a spiritual person and my family and I have always been in church and in a time like this your spiritual hope is really the only thing that you have to rely on. You can't rely on the government, it's just knowing that everything's going to be OK, you just have to have that faith to know that God is there, He's watching over everything that's happening, giving us the strength to endure what we have to endure until things get better.

Staff: I am confident that everything in my life has been led by the Lord for a reason, so there's no regret at all, any of it.

The sixth HHI item "I feel scared about my future." There are 19 interviews with 75 references. Of those, 8 interviews and 34 references come from volunteers, 4 interviews with 16 references from residents, and 7 interviews with 25 references from staff. Examples of those data include the following:

Volunteer: Just scared for them; scared for the city of New Orleans; scared for what's going to happen if someone doesn't get down there and start getting people out of those trailers.

Resident: We're kind of stressed. We have to be out of this hotel but we don't have the utilities hooked up. I don't know what we're going to do.

Staff: I said, "I'm scared, Lord. I don't know what's going to happen."

The seventh HHI item is "I can recall happy/joyful times" and is represented in 22 interviews and 57 references. Of those, 10 interviews with 23 references were from volunteers, 5 interviews with 16 references from residents, and 7 interviews with 18 references from staff. Examples of the references/data are as follows:

> Volunteer: I remember, we had some crazy guys on our team. We were on one of our breaks, drinking Gatorade, and the boys start dancing. They were trying to get us all to dance and we don't really dance (laughter), so it was just funny; we just laughed a lot. You know, you gotta have fun.

> Resident: We had an attic and I forgot I had some things in the attic and they [volunteers] went up there and they found some pictures and I was just so grateful that they found them and they were so happy that they found a few things for us.

> Staff: My first encounter of a homeowner was an 83-year-old lady. She just sat on her swing while she watched the group work. I'd talk with her and she told me about her garden and it was like she could see it and I'm seeing brown shrubs and a tree. A tree was in the middle of her house. There was nothing in bloom, there was nothing, none of her statues were there, but she could see it and she had such a positive attitude. She knew I was going to be getting married and she was telling me about a statue she had called "young love."

The eighth HHI item is "I have deep inner strength." Forty references in 17 interviews support this item, including 7 interviews with 15 references from volunteers, 5 interviews and 11 references from residents, and 5 interviews with 14 references from staff. Sample data are presented below:

> Volunteer: When you see someone in so much pain you just want to feel that with them, you don't want them to be alone in a dark place, you want to be able to come with them, set next to them and cry, and say you're not alone. I don't know what you've been through and no I can't ever feel the same way you do because I didn't ever go through your experience, but I'm going to set here and I'm going to cry with you.

> Resident: Katrina was like a dream; it wasn't my reality because of the peace I had within me. It didn't affect me as some. And then, when I saw "God is still here" on the car, it was like YES, I'm not crazy.

> Staff: I think more than anything it was just within myself, you know. The naiveté stopped, the self-consciousness stopped; the fact that I may not have felt qualified for any of the stuff I was doing for the past 2 months, all that stopped and I realized that the Lord had placed me here for a reason and I know what to do. He has shown me what to do and He has prepared me for this over the past 10 years of my life.

The ninth HHI item is "I am able to give and receive caring/love" with support from 145 references in 23 interviews. Of these, 9 interviews and 10 references come from volunteers, 5 interviews and 56 references from residents, and 9 interviews and 70 references from staff. Examples of data from each of these groups include the following:

> Volunteer: We were there to love them and to show them that we haven't forgotten about them and yeah, maybe we weren't down there restoring homes but we were down there restoring hearts. We love them and we want to hear about their story.

> Resident: I did take pictures of their names they wrote on my wall. I plan to print it out and get a big frame and hang it on my wall once I get back in my house. That way their names will be hanging on my wall so anyone that comes in and looks at the picture and see all these names will be "What's all this?" and I'm like, this is all the love that was given, shown with the redoing of my house.

Staff: She had such a feeling in the beginning of being out of her place because she was from another faith and I think it was such an awakening for her that these people loved her because she was herself (tearing, voice breaking), you know, not because she was a member of a particular faith.

The 10th HHI is "I have a sense of direction" with 145 references in 25 interviews. Eleven interviews and 56 references are from volunteers, 5 interviews and 26 references from residents, and 9 interviews and 64 references from staff. Sample data are provided below:

Volunteer: We asked him what do you want us to do, and what do you want us to bring? The distribution center gave us a general list of things to bring? When we got down there he already had 4 homes lined up ready to go.
Resident: I never had inner thoughts of leaving, just coming back and building.
Staff: It was time for me to leave. It was time for all of us to leave because it was then time for the residents of New Orleans [to step up]. You guys did everything you could do. You've done your gob. It's time. You can leave. And she [New Orleans official] told me that and I was just one happy camper. I just walked out of there. I said, "God put me here. I did whatever He wanted me to do and God just told me I could leave now."

The 11th HHI item "I believe that each day has potential" with 14 interviews and 21 references. Of those, volunteers account for 6 interviews and 7 references, residents with 4 interviews and 6 references, leaving 4 interviews and 8 references from staff. Three references, one per participant group, are provided:

Volunteer: I think there's hope, kind of like a renewing in that city. So much was damaged and yet the city now has a chance to kind of start over again.
Resident: I always look at people for the better part of them, even if they're on drugs and if I get to pass two to three words with them, you know you can be better, you know, that be my words to them, you CAN be better and I'll tell them, think about it.
Staff: She told me, "You guys came in and helped us, lifted our spirits, you did all this sort of thing. Now it's our turn. We need to do this now."

The final HHI is "I feel my life has value and worth" with 154 references in 23 interviews. Of these, 52 references in 11 volunteer interviews, 40 references in 4 resident interviews, and 62 references in 8 staff interviews. Examples of data supporting this item are reported below:

Volunteer: … just the appreciation, anytime we did something they were verbally very appreciative of us. It couldn't have made us feel any more important than they did.
Resident: This is your purpose. It's not about yourself, it's not even about giving money, [it's about] just being there and just providing your services.
Staff: I really felt this was an opportunity to impact lives, to really help people in their self-exploration, but you know, it turned by all the residents and volunteers I've met, I've been so blessed. I've received a tremendous reward from people I was trying to serve.

DISCUSSION

Through triangulation of the data, analysis revealed hope is present in the experience of all faith-based disaster response groups: volunteers, staff, and residents, despite the catastrophic devastation and personal sacrifices to respond or receive services. One explanation may be the specific activities or work of the response. In order for any of the work to occur, planning around very definitive goals was necessary. The goals provided a sense of direction; a place to start in what was otherwise an overwhelming sea of circumstances. Participants were willing to do the work because they saw potential and possibilities it created for the residents and city. Progress toward goals was immediate and long term; it required unified/joint efforts to accomplish. In working together, strong relationships were forged, leaving participants feeling they offered and received love. Even when circumstances were difficult and painful, the work and relationships provided a sense of joy and fun that gave participants pleasure in recounting.

Participants found comfort in their faith, a spiritual faith rarely referred to as a religious affiliation; this is consistent with the concept of spirituality found in nursing literature.[12–20] Participant's faith and deep inner strength gave them the fortitude to continue in the face of difficulty.

The worth and value of life were most frequently expressed as the work performed and the impact that work had on others. Involvement in the response provided purpose for the workers. The work was their calling, and by fulfilling the calling, their life had worth and value. It did not matter if the participants knew each other before, during, after, or never during the experience.

A Model of Faith-Based Disaster Response was proposed by Persell[8] with a context of Divine Agency.[21–23] A general awareness of the disaster and need was present before any participant engaged in faith-based disaster response. A time came when participants decided to offer or accept assistance. Strangers came together (Stranger-to-Stranger Interaction) and became involved in each other's lives such that pain (Social Suffering) and joy were willingly shared and deep relationships were forged.[24–26] Many of those relationships were still referred to as family (Communitas) years after the response.[27–31] Continual questioning and wondering about the process, people, and the work occurred (Reflection). Participants spoke of how their lives were changed (Transformation).[32] The validity of the HHI is confirmed in the qualitative data. The items align with the original model, as demonstrated in **Fig. 6**.

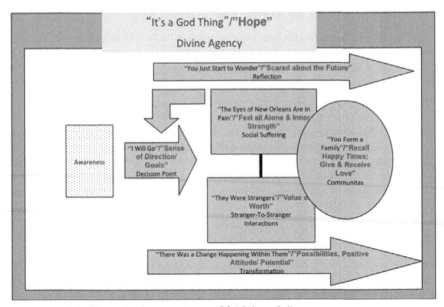

Fig. 6. A model of hope in the experience of faith-based disaster response.

SUMMARY

The following conclusions are proposed: (1) the theoretic underpinnings of hope are evident in faith-based disaster response, including hope as a life force; (2) the HHI is a valid measure of hope within the context of faith-based disaster response; (3) hope is embedded within faith-based disaster response; (4) faith-based disaster response is an intervention in hope; and (5) results of an intervention based on hope can last beyond 6 months as one study previously reported.[9]

An obvious limitation of this study is the sample of a single FBO. Additional limitations are the single geographic setting and singular disaster.

Additional research is indicated to determine if the same findings will be demonstrated in a variety of settings, types of disasters, and FBOs. The research question, yet to be answered, is whether all disaster response (faith-based, nongovernment organization, government, or other) is a vehicle of hope.

REFERENCES

1. United States House of Representatives Select Bipartisan Committee to Investigate the Preparation for and Response to Hurricane Katrina. A Failure of Initiative: final Report of the Select Bipartisan Committee to Investigate the Preparation for and the Response to Hurricane Katrina. Available at: http://katrina.house.gov/. Accessed February 15, 2006.
2. United States White House. The federal response to Hurricane Katrina: lessons learned. 2006. Available at: http://www.whitehouse.gov/reports/katrina-lessons-learned/. Accessed March 1, 2006.
3. National Volunteer Organizations Active in Disaster, Incorporated. NVOAD National Organization Members. 2014. Available at: http://www.nvoad.org/voad-network/national-members/. Accessed January 20, 2007.
4. Benzein E, Saveman B-I. One step towards the understanding of hope: a concept analysis. Int J Nurs Stud 1998;35:322–9.
5. Dufault K, Martocchio B. Hope: its spheres and dimensions. Nurs Clin North America 1985;20(2):379–91.
6. Herth KA, Cutcliffe JR. The concept of hope in nursing 6: research/education/policy/practice. Br J Nurs 2002;11(21):1404–11.
7. Wang CH. Developing a concept of hope from a human science perspective. Nurs Sci Q 2000;13(3):248–51.
8. Persell D. The lived experience of faith-based disaster response: a qualitative and quantitative analysis. Dissertation. Knoxville (TN): University of Tennessee; Hodges Library; 2008.
9. Rustoen T, Hanestad B. Nursing intervention to increase hope in cancer patients. J Clin Nurs 1998;7(1):19–27.
10. Tollett J, Thomas SP. A theory-based nursing intervention to instill hope in homeless veterans. Adv Nurs Sci 1995;18(2):76–90.
11. Snyder C. Conceptualizing, measuring, and nurturing hope. J Couns Development 1995;73:355–60.
12. Harden MG. Towards a faith-based program theory: a reconceptualization of program theory. Eval Rev 2006;30(4):481–504.
13. Miner-Williams D. Putting a puzzle together: making spirituality meaningful for nursing using an evolving theoretical framework. J Clin Nurs 2006;15(7):811–21.
14. Swinton J, McSherry W. Editorial: critical reflections on the current state of spirituality-in-nursing. J Clin Nurs 2006;15(7):801–2.

15. Clarke N. Transformational development as a valid strategy for use in the development of post-tsunami Aceh, Indonesia: the case of two Christian faith-based organizations. Transformation 2006;23(3):187–92.
16. McSherry W. The principal components model: a model for advancing spirituality and spiritual care within nursing and health care practice. J Clin Nurs 2006;15(7): 905–17.
17. Ross L. Spiritual care in nursing: an overview of the research to date. J Clin Nurs 2006;15(7):852–62.
18. Walter T. Spirituality in palliative care: opportunity or burden? Palliat Med 2002;16: 133–9.
19. Narayanasamy A. A review of spirituality as applied to nursing. Int J Nurs Stud 1999;36:117–25.
20. Ai A, Tice T, Peterson C, et al. Prayers, spiritual support and positive attitudes in coping with the September 11 national crisis. J Personal 2005;73(3):763–91.
21. Schwobel C. Divine agency and providence. Mod Theology 1987;3(3):225–44.
22. Yong A. On divine presence and divine agency: toward a foundational pneumatology. Asian J Pentecostal Stud 2000;3(2):167–88.
23. Henderson EH. Austin Farrer and D.Z. Phillips on lived faith, prayer and divine reality. Mod Theology 1985;1(3):223–43.
24. Wilkinson I. Health, risk and "social suffering". Health Risk Soc 2006;8(1):108.
25. Long ET. Suffering and transcendence. Int J Philos Religion 2006;60:139–48.
26. Dossa P. "Witnessing" social suffering: testimonial narratives of women from Afghanistan. Br Columbia Stud 2005;147:27–49.
27. Turner V. The ritual process: structure and anti-structure. Chicago: Aldine; 1969.
28. Turner V. Dramas, fields and metaphors: action in human society. Ithaca (NY): Cornell University Press; 1974.
29. Turner V. From ritual to theater: the human seriousness of play. New York: Performing Arts Journal Publications; 1982.
30. Sharpe EK. Delivering communitas: wilderness adventure and the making of community. J Leis Res 2005;37(3):255–80.
31. Spencer J, Hersch G, Aldridge J, et al. Daily life and forms of "communitas" in a personal care home for elders. Res Aging 2001;23(6):611–32.
32. Sugden C. Transformational development: current state of understanding and practice. Transformational Development 2003;20(2):70–6.
33. Miller JF. Development of an instrument to measure hope. Nurs Res 1988;37(1): 6–10.
34. Nowotny M. Assessment of hope in patients with cancer: development of an instrument. Oncol Nurs Forum 1989;16(1):57–61.
35. Herth K. Development and refinement of an instrument to measure hope. Sch Inq Nurs Pract 1991;5(1):39–51.
36. Herth K. Abbreviated instrument to measure hope: development and psychometric evaluation. J Adv Nurs 1992;17:1251–9.
37. Raleigh EH, Boehm S. Development of the multidimensional hope scale. J Nurs Meas 1994;2(2):155–67.
38. Snyder CR. Conceptualizing, measuring, and nurturing hope. J Couns Dev 1995; 73:355–60.
39. Snyder CR, Sympson SC, Ybasco FC, et al. Development and validation of the state of hope scale. J Pers Soc Psychol 1996;70:321–5.
40. Snyder CR. The development and validation of the children's hope scale. J Pediatr Psychol 1997;22(3):399–421.

41. Dubrov A. The influence of hope, openness to experience and situational control on resistance to organizational change. MA thesis. Department of Psychology, Bar-Ilan University. 2002.
42. Hendricks CS, Hendricks D, Murdaugh C, et al. Psychometric testing of the miller hope scale with rural southern adolescents. J Multicult Nurs Health 2005;11(3): 41–50.
43. Marques S, Pais-Ribeiro JL, Lopez SJ. Validation of a portuguese version of the children's hope scale. Sch Psychol Int 2009;30(5):538–51.
44. Arnau RC, Martinez PM, Guzman I, et al. A Spanish-language versioin of the Herth Hope Scale: development and psychometric evaluation in a Peruvian Sample. Educ Psychol Meas 2010;1–17.
45. Bernardo A. Extending hope theory: Internal and external locus of trait hope. Pers Individ Dif 2010;49(8):944–9.
46. Gestel-Timmermans H, van den Bogarrd J, Brouwers E, et al. Hope as a determinant of mental health recovery: a psychometric evaluation of the herth hope index-Dutch version. Scand J Caring Sci 2010;24:67–74.
47. Schrank B, Woppmann A, Sibitz I, et al. Development and validation of an integrative scale to assess hope. Health Expect 2011;14(4):417–28.
48. Chan KS, Li HC, Chan W, et al. Herth hope index: psychometric testing of the Chinese version. J Adv Nurs 2012;68(9):2079–85.
49. Ripamonti CI, Buonaccorso L, Maruelli A, et al. Hope herth index (HHI): a validation study in Italian patients with solid and hematological malignancies on active cancer treatment. Tumori 2012;98:385–92.
50. Dew-Reeves SE, Athay MM, Kelley SD. Validation and use of the Children's Hope Scale-Revised PTPB Edition/(CHS-PTPB): High initial youth hope and elevated baseline symptomatology predict poor treatment outcomes. Adm Policy Ment Health 2012;39:60–70.

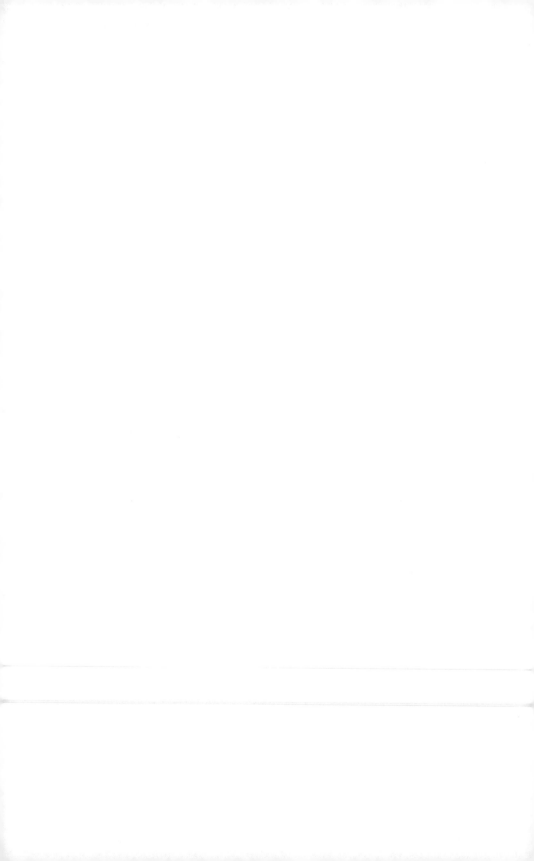

Index

Note: Page numbers of article titles are in **boldface** type.

A

American Nurses Credentialing Center, development of National Healthcare Disaster Certification by, 565

American Red Cross, model for identifying client needs in disaster shelter, **647–662**

Appalachia, FEMA response to emergency in, **599–611**

B

Behavioral health, of US military nurses responding to disasters, 619–620

C

California, wildfires in, nurses' role in, 636–637

Centers for Medicare and Medicaid Services, regulatory requirements of, and emergency preparedness, 553

Certification, development of National Healthcare Disaster Certification by American Nurses Credentialing Center, 565

Chemical removal, hospital decontamination, **663–674**

Chemical Stockpile Emergency Preparedness Program, 547–551

CMIST program, identifying client needs in disaster shelter, 653–656

Coalitions. *See* Health care coalitions.

Communication issues, for US military nurses serving in disaster response, 620–621

Competencies, disaster-specific nursing, 556–558. 559–561

    agency, 557–558

    education and training to meet, 558

    in the National Disaster Health Consortium, 558–564

    specialty, 556–557

Contamination, hospital decontamination, **663–674**

    radiation exposure, fear and patient care adaptations for, **675–695**

Cot-to-Cot program, identifying client needs in disaster shelter, 653–656

D

Decontamination, hospital, **663–674**

    best practices, 668–672

    current state of, 664–665

    implications for first receivers, 665–668

Disaster preparedness, implications for nursing, 555–721

    development of health care coalitions for, **545–554**

        Centers for Medicare and Medicaid Services regulatory requirements, 553

        Chemical Stockpile Emergency Preparedness Program, 547–551

        current status of, 551–552

UNITED STATES POSTAL SERVICE — Statement of Ownership, Management, and Circulation (All Periodicals Publications Except Requester Publications)

1. Publication Title	2. Publication Number	3. Filing Date
NURSING CLINICS OF NORTH AMERICA	598 – 960	9/18/2016

4. Issue Frequency	5. Number of Issues Published Annually	6. Annual Subscription Price
MAR, JUN, SEP, DEC	4	$150.00

7. Complete Mailing Address of Known Office of Publication (Not printer) (Street, city, county, state, and ZIP+4®)
ELSEVIER INC.
360 PARK AVENUE SOUTH
NEW YORK, NY 10010-1710

Contact Person
STEPHEN R. BUSHING
Telephone (include area code)
215-239-3688

8. Complete Mailing Address of Headquarters or General Business Office of Publisher (Not printer)
ELSEVIER INC.
360 PARK AVENUE SOUTH
NEW YORK, NY 10010-1710

9. Full Names and Complete Mailing Addresses of Publisher, Editor, and Managing Editor (Do not leave blank)

Publisher (Name and complete mailing address)
ADRIANNE BRIGIDO, ELSEVIER INC.
1600 JOHN F KENNEDY BLVD. SUITE 1800
PHILADELPHIA, PA 19103-2899

Editor (Name and complete mailing address)
KERRY HOLLAND, ELSEVIER INC.
1600 JOHN F KENNEDY BLVD. SUITE 1800
PHILADELPHIA, PA 19103-2899

Managing Editor (Name and complete mailing address)
PATRICK MANLEY, ELSEVIER INC.
1600 JOHN F KENNEDY BLVD. SUITE 1800
PHILADELPHIA, PA 19103-2899

10. Owner (Do not leave blank. If the publication is owned by a corporation, give the name and address of the corporation immediately followed by the names and addresses of all stockholders owning or holding 1 percent or more of the total amount of stock. If not owned by a corporation, give the names and addresses of the individual owners. If owned by a partnership or other unincorporated firm, give its name and address as well as those of each individual owner. If the publication is published by a nonprofit organization, give its name and address.)

Full Name	Complete Mailing Address
WHOLLY OWNED SUBSIDIARY OF REED/ELSEVIER, US HOLDINGS	1600 JOHN F KENNEDY BLVD. SUITE 1800 PHILADELPHIA, PA 19103-2899

11. Known Bondholders, Mortgagees, and Other Security Holders Owning or Holding 1 Percent or More of Total Amount of Bonds, Mortgages, or Other Securities. If none, check box ► ☐ None

Full Name	Complete Mailing Address
N/A	

12. Tax Status (For completion by nonprofit organizations authorized to mail at nonprofit rates) (Check one)
The purpose, function, and nonprofit status of this organization and the exempt status for federal income tax purposes:
☐ Has Not Changed During Preceding 12 Months
☐ Has Changed During Preceding 12 Months (Publisher must submit explanation of change with this statement)

13. Publication Title	14. Issue Date for Circulation Data Below
NURSING CLINICS OF NORTH AMERICA	JUNE 2016

PS Form **3526**, July 2014 (Page 1 of 4 (see instructions page 4)) PSN: 7530-01-000-9931 PRIVACY NOTICE: See our privacy policy on www.usps.com

15. Extent and Nature of Circulation			Average No. Copies Each Issue During Preceding 12 Months	No. Copies of Single Issue Published Nearest to Filing Date
a. Total Number of Copies (Net press run)			862	853
b. Paid Circulation (By Mail and Outside the Mail)	(1)	Mailed Outside-County Paid Subscriptions Stated on PS Form 3541 (Include paid distribution above nominal rate, advertiser's proof copies, and exchange copies)	481	486
	(2)	Mailed In-County Paid Subscriptions Stated on PS Form 3541 (Include paid distribution above nominal rate, advertiser's proof copies, and exchange copies)	0	0
	(3)	Paid Distribution Outside the Mails Including Sales Through Dealers and Carriers, Street Vendors, Counter Sales, and Other Paid Distribution Outside USPS®	148	158
	(4)	Paid Distribution by Other Classes of Mail Through the USPS (e.g. First-Class Mail®)	0	0
c. Total Paid Distribution (Sum of 15b (1), (2), (3), and (4))			629	644
d. Free or Nominal Rate Distribution (By Mail and Outside the Mail)	(1)	Free or Nominal Rate Outside-County Copies included on PS Form 3541	20	64
	(2)	Free or Nominal Rate In-County Copies Included on PS Form 3541	0	0
	(3)	Free or Nominal Rate Copies Mailed at Other Classes Through the USPS (e.g. First-Class Mail)	0	0
	(4)	Free or Nominal Rate Distribution Outside the Mail (Carriers or other means)	0	0
e. Total Free or Nominal Rate Distribution (Sum of 15d (1), (2), (3) and (4))			20	64
f. Total Distribution (Sum of 15c and 15e)			649	708
g. Copies not Distributed (See Instructions to Publishers #4 (page #3))			213	145
h. Total (Sum of 15f and g)			862	853
i. Percent Paid (15c divided by 15f times 100)			97%	91%

* If you are claiming electronic copies, go to line 16 on page 3. If you are not claiming electronic copies, skip to line 17 on page 3.

PS Form **3526**, July 2014 (Page 2 of 4)

16. Electronic Copy Circulation	Average No. Copies Each Issue During Preceding 12 Months	No. Copies of Single Issue Published Nearest to Filing Date
a. Paid Electronic Copies ►	0	0
b. Total Paid Print Copies (Line 15c) + Paid Electronic Copies (Line 16a) ►	629	644
c. Total Print Distribution (Line 15f) + Paid Electronic Copies (Line 16a) ►	649	708
d. Percent Paid (Both Print & Electronic Copies) (16b divided by 16c × 100) ►	97%	91%

☒ I certify that 50% of all my distributed copies (electronic and print) are paid above a nominal price.

17. Publication of Statement of Ownership
☒ If the publication is a general publication, publication of this statement is required. Will be printed in the DECEMBER 2016 issue of this publication. ☐ Publication not required.

18. Signature and Title of Editor, Publisher, Business Manager, or Owner

STEPHEN R. BUSHING - INVENTORY DISTRIBUTION CONTROL MANAGER   Date 9/18/2016

I certify that all information furnished on this form is true and complete. I understand that anyone who furnishes false or misleading information on this form or who omits material or information requested on the form may be subject to criminal sanctions (including fines and imprisonment) and/or civil sanctions (including civil penalties).

PS Form **3526**, July 2014 (Page 3 of 4) PRIVACY NOTICE: See our privacy policy on www.usps.com

Edwards Brothers Malloy
Ann Arbor MI. USA
December 5, 2016

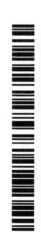